Where Does My Horse Hurt?

A Hands-On Guide to Evaluating Pain and Dysfunction Using Chiropractic Methods

Renee Tucker, DVM

Certified in Equine Chiropractic and Acupuncture

Photographs by Ginger-Kathleen Coombs

Illustrations by Patty Capps

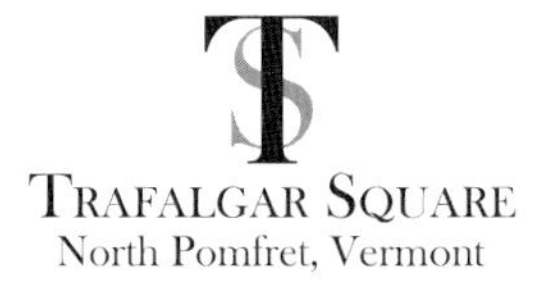

Trafalgar Square
North Pomfret, Vermont

First published in 2011 by
Trafalgar Square Books
North Pomfret, Vermont 05053

Printed in China

Disclaimer of Liability

The author and publisher shall have neither liability nor responsibility to any person or entity with respect to any loss or damage caused or alleged to be caused directly or indirectly by the information contained in this book. While the book is as accurate as the author can make it, there may be errors, omissions, and inaccuracies.

Library of Congress Cataloging-in-Publication Data

Tucker, Renee.
Where does my horse hurt? : a hands-on guide to evaluating pain and dysfunction using chiropractic methods / Renee Tucker.
p. cm.
Includes bibliographical references and index.
ISBN 978-1-57076-486-8
1. Horses—Wounds and injuries—Chiropractic treatment. 2. Horses—Wounds and injuries—Diagnosis. I. Title.
SF951.T83 2011
636.1'089—dc22
2011006203

Book design by Lauryl Eddlemon
Cover design by RM Didier
Typefaces: Minion, Myriad

10 9 8 7 6 5 4

To all my cherished clients, especially those who said, "If only I had known."

Contents

Foreword

BY DR. JOYCE HARMAN

If you are a horse owner who wants your horse to always feel his best, or you have a horse with a "mystery lameness," you have probably searched all over for answers. And in the process you have heard theories, been promised cures, and may have spent a considerable amount of money pursuing solutions.

As a horse owner in this modern era, you need to be in charge of your horse's medical care. Ideally you have a team of professionals you can trust to help you make decisions, but in many cases, they may not have all the answers. Or, maybe you live in an area with limited professional help and need to know what types of treatments to pursue. Perhaps your own health and well-being has been improved by chiropractic care, and you now wonder if it could also help your horse.

No matter what your reasons are for picking up this book, Dr. Renee Tucker has written an excellent resource that can guide you through a complete physical examination of your horse's musculoskeletal system. The pictures and anatomical drawings are very clear and make it possible for *anyone* to accomplish these examinations. She details how to perform an exam of each joint and how to keep safe while doing it, so neither you nor your horse gets hurt.

Using this book, you will get to know your horse in a way you never have before, and you will also learn to notice when something has changed. In many cases your horse comes in from the paddock (after a long night of "partying" with his buddies in the mud)a bit "off," and you have no idea what actually happened. All you know is that he does not feel or move quite right. A thorough exam following the instructions in this book will not tell you how he did it, but it *will* help you decide what body parts are involved and guide you as to the next best step for helping him.

Dr. Tucker has included very useful checklists in each section of the book to help you decide what symptoms might link to your findings and what treatments might be the best to pursue—that is, do you need a veterinarian, a chiropractor, a farrier, a saddle fitter, or all of the above?

This is one of those books that should be on every horse owner's shelf; in reality, it should not sit on the shelf, it should be in the barn and get used on a regular basis. It does not matter what sport you pursue with your horse, or if your horse is mostly retired, or if you just ride occasionally for pleasure—this book will help you be a much better educated horse owner.

Joyce Harman, DVM, MRCVS

Author of *The Horse's Pain-Free Back and Saddle-Fit Book, The Western Horse's Pain-Free Back and Saddle-Fit Book, English Saddles: How to Fit—Pain-Free (DVD)*, and *Western Saddles: How to Fit—Pain-Free (DVD)*
www.harmanyequine.com

PREFACE

How We Are Going to Change the World

In this world of ours, a lot of things need changing. But when it all seems overwhelming, we can take heart by starting with just this one: Many, many horses are in pain, and the people responsible for their well-being usually don't even know it. Owners and riders find out when their horse develops a performance or lameness issue, but the problem—the root of the pain—is usually there long before it becomes obvious.

What's the one thing we do every day before we ride? The one thing we always do? We pick out the horse's feet. Why do we do that? Because we know, "No foot, no horse." That is one of the first lessons we learn and often the first we pass along to new riders. In terms of the horse's well-being, "No foot, no horse" is an absolute truth.

But what about the horse's back? Or head? Or ribs? Are they not just as integral to the horse's movement and ability to perform? Wouldn't it be wonderful if we could determine if these other parts of the horse hurt or are not functioning right with a quick, daily exam, much like our general analysis of the horse's feet when we clean them? Well, it would be—and can be! That's what this book is for: It is a way for anyone to learn how, in only five to ten minutes, he or she can check over the horse's entire body and then know that the horse is doing well (he is free from pain or discomfort, and his movement is optimal), or that an area of his body needs to be watched or an apparent problem addressed.

This book is designed for every person who cares for and about horses. Whether you are a horse owner, veterinarian, farrier, trainer, massage therapist (or specialist in another form of bodywork), show judge, or the mom or dad who does the grooming and pays the bills, you can learn to check the horse in your life for pain and potential problems. Then you can pass this information on to your friends, barn-mates, students, clients, and children...and slowly but surely the horse's world will indeed be changed.

This book *does not* attempt to teach you how to adjust your horse. This book *does* teach you how to know when your horse would benefit from a chiropractic adjustment. This book *does not* teach you how to be a veterinarian. But it *does* teach you how to find the places where your horse is hurting (even when it is not obviously hot or swollen). The direct result is you will be better informed and better able to work with your veterinarian as together you try to alleviate the source of your horse's pain.

I must also note that this book also does not address every single possible reason for horses to suffer from pain, discomfort, and inhibited movement. For example, I assume that you know that poor riding itself can cause pain. As there are already many excellent books on riding technique, I have excluded that from the discussion.

You will be amazed by how much you will learn about your horse by using the simple tools in this book. You will maximize your ability to detect small changes in your horse from day to day. And you will celebrate when you detect and resolve a problem at an early stage, therefore eliminating the potential need for months of stall rest or expensive treatments at a later date. I am already excited about the success that is sure to be yours, and I sincerely hope you will email or write me (see my contact information on p. 165), and share your stories!

Thank you for joining me. You are going to love this because one day you will be able to say that you were a part of changing the horse world from the beginning.

RENEE TUCKER, DVM

Certified in Equine Chiropractic
and Acupuncture

Acknowledgments

I'd like to acknowledge the people without whom this book would not exist. That was a tricky sentence, wasn't it? Anyway…

Thank you to everyone at Trafalgar Square Books for their hard work and belief in this book.

BIG THANKS to my dearest Sam-friend Lydia for all her help with my kids and computers, and all around encouragement and support.

Thanks to my friend Jesus from whom all true healing comes.

Thanks to my dad for his nonstop help, even when overwhelmed, and for being proud of me even before this book was finished.

Thanks to Merrilee Asla Lee for her work with photos and editing and dinners. Thanks also to Dick Lee for his editing and support. Merrilee offers lovely pictures and greeting cards for sale and a portion of the proceeds goes to helping animals. You can contact her at merrilee3@msn.com.

Thanks to Patty Capps for her astronomical effort in making the illustrations perfect. And for her patience with my nit-picking. And her hilarious emails. She can be contacted at equinemity@live.com.

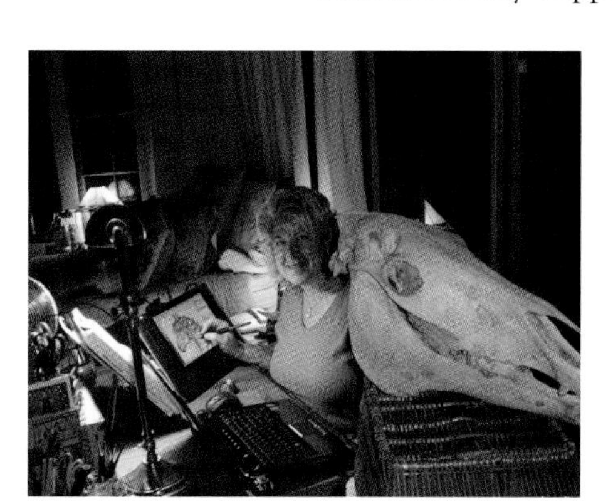

Patty Capps, the illustrator, hard at work in her "lair."

Thanks to Ginger-Kathleen Coombs, the amazing and talented photographer. She can be reached at elijahparkphotography.com.

Thanks to Katherine Tilken of Short Acre Farms in Hockinson, Washington, who generously allowed the photographs to be taken on her beautiful property.

Thanks to the horse models and their owners. You look great!

Special thanks to R.W. Henry, DVM, PhD (my professor of anatomy at the University of Tennessee, Knoxville—now almost 20 years ago!) who so graciously proofed the anatomic illustrations for correctness.

To all my clients, whom I consider to be my friends and family: Thanks for being my "guinea pigs." Ha! Just kidding! You're not guinea pigs. I love you! You are all great and I am honored to be part of your horse's health team.

And, lastly, to Milton and Roady, the "Roadmaster."

PART ONE

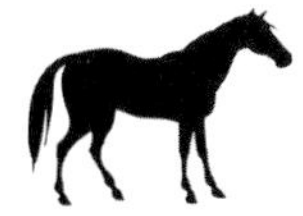

Introduction to Chiropractic and Body Checkups

CHAPTER 1
A Chiropractic Awakening

Introduction

I practiced veterinary medicine for five years before discovering the invaluable benefits chiropractic can offer our horses—both those used for recreation and those competed at any level. I was amazed by the difference an adjustment (or adjustments) could make in the physical and mental well-being of the horse. You see, so many of our horses "hurt"—whether a sharp pain or a dull ache, whether in a physical sense or an emotional one, whether as obvious as a buck or rear, or as subtle as a minute decrease in a limb's range of motion. And it is not only in the owner's best interest to cure what ails her riding partner because of the potential of improved performance, it is also usually her greatest wish to keep her horse comfortable, free of pain, and happy when at ease and when in motion.

This inspired me to go back to school and become a certified animal chiropractor (I tell more of my story, beginning on p. 4).

Over the 10 years I have now spent adjusting horses with hundreds of different symptoms brought on by a vast range of causes, it has become very clear to me that owners would benefit from being able to determine, in a quick and simple way, whether or not their horse's problem (or problems) could be solved by a visit from a chiropractor, whether they really need to consult the veterinarian, or if another qualified professional might not be a better choice for an accurate diagnosis with the least amount of time and money spent. Why should owners be able to do this? Because often a 20-minute session with a chiropractor can resolve an issue that might take countless (expensive) visits from a veterinarian to diagnose, if he is able to diagnose the problem at all. Because thousands of horses are sold, retired, or otherwise "given up on" every year due to behavior problems, physical issues, and mystery lamenesses that no amount of money, time, or medicine can cure, usually because the wrong horse care professional was consulted at the wrong time (if anyone was consulted at all).

It is my goal to help you, help your horse remain free of discomfort and pain, and enjoy the full range of movement of which his magnificent body is capable. I can do this by teaching you 27 easy Body Checkups, or ways to diagnose the source of your horse's pain or discomfort. This book is *not* intended to teach you chiropractic technique; it is meant as a sensible plan of action for maintaining your horse's physical health and general happiness while preserving your sanity and your pocketbook.

Your horse's body "talks" to you in countless ways, and the pages ahead tell you what it is saying.

What Happened One Day

"I can always tell when my horse's rib goes 'out' because he gets irritable and lays his ears back at me," said this supposedly competent and knowledgeable horsewoman. But, now I knew the truth. She was missing a few marbles!

I kept a straight face. And I even asked her which rib was out. She pushed on one of them and said, "See? See how he doesn't like that?" I was thinking, "Hmmm. I wouldn't like being poked in the side either."

At the time, I was a traditional equine veterinarian. I had graduated vet school from the University of Tennessee in 1995, and what I'd mostly heard from my professors was that chiropractic was pure "quackery."

But then this woman asked me whom I'd recommend as a chiropractor for her horse. And, since this "Who do you recommend as an equine chiropractor?" question had been coming up more frequently in my practice, I realized I was going to have to figure out the truth about chiropractic, and maybe even find out first hand.

My apologies to those of you who have always known the benefits of chiropractic care. I had never gone to a chiropractor. And I hadn't known anyone who had visited one either. If you recall, about 15 years ago (or more), chiropractors were an object of ridicule on television.

I decided to attend the only animal chiropractic school that existed in 1998: Options for Animals in Moline, Illinois, affiliated with the American Veterinary Chiropractic Association (AVCA). In order to go to this school, you have to be either a veterinarian or a chiropractor. This means that you already have a doctorate in medicine. Because of the students' medical background, the teachers don't have to go over basic anatomy, physiology, neurology.

The school teaches in "modules." There are six modules you must attend to become certified in animal chiropractic. Each module comprises five, twelve-hour, intensive days. Then you go home for a few weeks—practicing what you've learned—to return the following month for exams and another intensive five days. The last module is five days of written and skills tests. *If* you pass, and not everyone does, then you are certified in animal chiropractic. Technically, you cannot call yourself an "animal chiropractor"—you can only say you are "certified in animal chiropractic (CAC)." I tend to lapse and use the term "animal chiropractor" because it is easier to say.

I was probably the most skeptical person in our full class of 60 students. I pretended not to be. And I pretended to understand what they were talking about. Oh, I understood the words. But the "light bulb" didn't go off for me until the third module. I did try. It's just that chiropractic is extremely difficult to explain to someone who has never experienced it, or even seen it done.

I learned that we humans (and horses) have an intricate series of mechanisms that compensate when something in our body goes out of *its normal alignment* (see Compensation, p. 14). For example, say you sleep "funny" and tweak your neck. When you get up, your body's first priority is to make sure your eyes are horizontal for *proprioception,* which means that you know where you are "in space." So that you don't walk around with your head tilted sideways, the body automatically releases some neck muscles, tightens others, and starts using the back and shoulder muscles to help with the neck. You have probably felt all this muscle action in the form of a "knot" above your shoulder blade.

The body can compensate like this for years; you don't feel any pain. It is only when it cannot compensate anymore that you start to notice a problem.

My First Chiropractor Visit

As I began to have some understanding of how chiropractic worked and how useful it might be, I thought to myself, "Well, you'd better go, at least once, to a chiropractor, so you can say you've gone. I mean, how will it look if you've never been to a chiropractor when you're adjusting someone's horse?" So I decided I'd go. Once.

I went to a chiropractor my landlady recommended. Normal looking office. Friendly receptionist. Then into the exam room walks a long-haired guy in clogs and a kilt. Now my blood pressure went up. The chiropractors in my animal chiropractic class had looked like regular people. I think this fellow noticed how my eyes were bugging out because he asked me lots of questions, and for a while, we chatted about the animal chiropractic school and chiropractic in general.

I got up off the table feeling loose and relaxed. My sacroiliac joints had been *out of alignment* (called "*subluxated*"—see p. 9) for so long that I hadn't even realized it was affecting my posture. The chiropractor told me this was why my lower back had been aching—it wasn't just because I was getting older. And, I *didn't* need to do more sit-ups to support my lower back! Hooray! As I had not been in any accidents, he just had me come to see him twice more, and then whenever I felt like it after that.

Well, I was really sold. I had gone to see this man with no idea anything was wrong with me, and now I felt 10 years younger. Many people have no idea something is wrong with their body, or that some part of it is out of alignment, thereby needing a chiropractic adjustment. It's only when they get an adjustment that they wish they had seen the chiro-

"She Just Feels Stiff…"

One time I was adjusting Mandy, a 12-year-old Quarter Horse mare, and I couldn't believe how badly this horse was out of alignment. Every joint needed fixing. "She just feels stiff," was all her owner had noticed. I always enquire whether there had been any recent falls, accidents, surgeries—or anything else—to get a complete picture of the horse's history. But Mandy hadn't had anything happen. I just couldn't believe it. I kept asking periodically, "Any slips in the mud?" "Did she pull back on the cross-ties?" "Fall in the trailer?" No. No. No.

Finally, toward the end of our session, Mandy's owner casually mentioned, "Well, about four years ago she did fall down that cliff, but she was fine."

Apparently, during a trail ride, the horse had somersaulted down a very steep incline for about 100 feet or so (the rider was thrown clear). Mandy was "fine" because she only had a few scratches and was able to be ridden back home. But now the owner was beginning to notice the consequences: Mandy's "compensation system" had been working so well she had appeared quite normal—despite all the subluxations I detected.

practor sooner! And it is the same with horses. Owners frequently don't recognize when their horse is out of alignment until behavior or lameness brings the issue to their attention.

Are You Sure This Isn't Quackery?

I really understand people who are of the opinion that animal chiropractic may be quackery. Why? Because that's what I had thought until about 1997! How can we know chiropractic works on animals? The animals can't talk.

Then I found out that the man credited with discovering chiropractic in the United States in 1895, D.D. Palmer, had a son, B.J., who wanted to make sure the results he and his father were getting with people were not caused by the placebo effect. He did extensive scientific testing of chiropractic on animals. His reasoning was simple—animals do not fake symptoms. And they also don't lie and tell you a treatment worked to make you feel good. Long story short, chiropractic works excellently on animals. (B.J. Palmer's research is available for review at Palmer Chiropractic College in Illinois.)

As a traditional equine veterinarian, I had always been fascinated by "mystery" cases, such as subtle lameness, intermittent soreness, or the—really challenging—"phantom" lameness. I enjoyed looking for clues for the causes, though very often, you can't find a specific answer without an MRI, and most owners can't afford this diagnostic tool. But when I added chiropractic to my repertoire of treatments, I was amazed how many of these cases had a chiropractic solution.

I remember being called to see a 17½-hand, four-year-old, bay Warmblood named Dualin. The owner and trainer told me right up front that I was their last resort. They were going to "put him out to pasture" if I couldn't find anything. Dualin's symptoms were quite unique. While trotting, he would be three-legged lame (holding one foot off the ground) for a minute, be head-bobbing lame for another few minutes until he warmed up, and then he would act fine. This lameness would occur in one front leg or the other and only with a saddle on (with or without a rider).

"But we've checked the saddle fit, had both front legs blocked up to the shoulder, complete X-rays, and a nuclear scan…and nothing!" said the owner. The poor woman was desperate to help her horse, and had already spent upward of $10,000.

I had never heard of anything like this in vet school, or even at the chiropractic school, for that matter. I said, "Well, I'll check him head to toe and see if there are any out-of-alignment issues I can fix." And, happy day! Dualin' had "ribs out" (the correct term is *subluxated,* see p. 9) behind both shoulder blades, right where his saddle was sitting.

It turns out this gigantic horse was something of a sissy, and his "lameness" was his way of showing his owner how his ribs hurt when the saddle was put on. Once his muscles warmed up and his brain acclimated to the saddle pressure on his ribs, he was able to work normally—in a way similar to us not noticing our clothes on our body after a few seconds. Once his ribs were adjusted—a one-time adjustment—he never showed this unusual lameness again.

My Misconceptions

I had always thought that chiropractic treatment was a fairly new field, but then I discovered that there are ancient Chinese (2700 BC) and Egyptian (4000 BC) manuscripts that describe chiropractic. And in 500 BC Hippocrates said, "Get knowledge of the spine, for this is the requisite for many diseases." So chiropractic has been around for thousands of years, not just a handful of decades.

I also had been lead to believe chiropractic had not been clinically proven. In fact, there are multiple scientific, peer-reviewed journals that show the science and benefits of chiropractic. There is no scientific reason to doubt that chiropractic treatments correct subluxations.

Yet another misconception I had was that once you start going to a chiropractor, you have to go to appointments forever or it doesn't work—that it's "just a money-making scheme." I'd heard this from someone who had gone to a chiropractor a couple times, but was dissatisfied. Since I didn't know any better at the time (and didn't care to find out), I filed this in my brain as a "truth." However, the real truth is that people often need multiple adjustments at first, especially if they have been in an accident. Once your alignment is correct, then you can go only as often as you want or need. Human chiropractic "maintenance" schedules range from "whenever" to "once a week." The best plan is the one that works for you.

There are no stupid questions, only ignorant assumptions, of which I have plenty to share. But having come from thinking "chiropractic is all quackery" to making chiropractic the focus of my veterinary practice (for over 10 years now), I can honestly tell you that it really works.

Unless you're off to the barn, I'll talk about how chiropractic works—in simple terms—in the next chapter.

CHAPTER 2

How Chiropractic Works

Subluxation

Before I attempt to explain how chiropractic works, I need to discuss the term "subluxation." Most importantly, you should know that a *medical* subluxation is not the same as a *chiropractic* subluxation. The word means one thing to a medical doctor and another to a chiropractor; consequently, there is some confusion about the word's usage.

MEDICAL SUBLUXATION

I'll explain the common use of the term in traditional medicine first. I'm sure you are familiar with a dislocated shoulder, for example, where the arm is completely out of the shoulder joint. A *medical* subluxation, simply put, is a dislocation that is *not* all the way out of the joint, and unlike the chiropractic condition, it can be seen by your doctor on X-ray.

CHIROPRACTIC SUBLUXATION

The practical *chiropractic* definition of a subluxation is that a joint is not working properly. It also may hurt the patient when you try to move the affected joint through its normal range of motion. This includes back joints as well as leg joints. A chiropractic subluxation is rarely visible on X-ray. A chiropractic subluxation actually has an even longer name, the *vertebral subluxation complex (VSC)*. The VSC includes the vertebra involved, plus a number of "behind-the-scenes" players such as pain; neural transmission dysfunction (i.e. nerves sending or receiving incorrect or slow signals); edema (swelling); adhesions (early scar tissue); and biochemical abnormalities.

So there is a lot going on underneath the surface of a subluxation. Because of the complexity involved, subluxated joints have a variety of symptoms. Some joints are completely "stuck" and don't move at all. Or, they only move in one direction but not another. Others are so stuck in one direction that the muscles have tightened around them and appear "rock hard." Or, joints appear to be fine, but as soon as you try to move them, the muscles "splint" around them to keep them from moving and to avoid pain. Whatever the signs are, if joints are not moving properly through their normal range of motion, they are "subluxated," in chiropractic terms.

Because "subluxation" is a very long word and "vertebral subluxation complex" even longer to say, instead many chiropractors use shorthand terminology and just say something is "out." (If you've been to a chiropractor, you know when your back is "out," and you know how much happier you are when it's back "in!") However, I generally use "subluxation" or "VSC" in this book, because they are the correct terms.

Okay. So far you know:

1) Chiropractic subluxations are *not* medical subluxations.
2) Chiropractic subluxations are officially called vertebral subluxation complexes (VSCs), which include the vertebra plus a number of "behind-the-scenes" players.
3) When a joint is not working properly through its entire range of motion, and/or there is pain (it "hurts") when you try to move the joint, it's likely a subluxation is causing the problem.

A subluxated joint means it is not working properly, and it may hurt the horse when you try to move the joint through its normal range of motion.

Joint Fluid Renewal System

Joint supplements are wonderful things. But allow me to let you in on a little secret—chiropractic care helps all of your horse's joints. Here's why: A joint needs to move in order to have healthy joint fluid; the old joint fluid is flushed out and new joint fluid brought in *only* when the joint moves.

As a human example, take someone with a broken ankle. Studies have shown that joints start to deteriorate after 12 hours in a cast. When the cast is removed, the ankle is extremely stiff. A lot of times physical therapy is needed to start getting the ankle to move again.

So when your horse's joints—whether they are leg or back joints—are subluxated, and therefore not moving properly, they are not getting all the joint fluid they need. Chiropractic care enables the joints to move through their entire range of motion, naturally regenerating joint fluid.

In the plainest words I can find, when you have a chiropractically subluxated joint, you have a joint that is not moving right, and it may hurt. This is something you want to fix. "Fixing" a VSC is called an "adjustment."

Adjustments

When a chiropractor comes out to "adjust" your horse, he or she will first perform an exam. During the exam, the chiropractor moves every joint through its normal range of motion to see if it is working properly.

Once a chiropractor has found a subluxation, the process of returning that joint to its normal ability to move is called an "adjustment." The American Veterinary Chiropractic Association definition of a chiropractic adjustment is: "A short-lever, high velocity, controlled thrust by hand or instrument that is directed at specific articulations to correct vertebral subluxations."

This description sounds very scientific, and it is. But what's really happening?

The chiropractor sends a signal—via the adjustment—to the body's innate healing mechanisms. This signal contains what is needed to fix the VSC. Because of the neural dysfunction involved, it's like the body's healing mechanisms have only been able to see the VSC in a fog, and therefore have been unable to correct it. The adjustment is like a sudden lightning flash whereby the body gets a glimpse of exactly what it needs to do to eliminate the VSC—which it does immediately.

The adjustment itself is simply a super-quick movement of the subluxated bone (spinal vertebra or leg bone) through its normal range of motion. This movement is so fast that it must be dead-on accurate with regards to angle, timing, and force. Sometimes a vertebra or leg bone is unable to be moved through its entire range of motion during the adjustment. Nevertheless the "flash signal" that the adjustment sends is still sufficient for the body to begin the healing process.

I'll quote here a paragraph about VSMT (Veterinary Spinal Manipulative Therapy) from the book *Recognizing the Horse in Pain…and What You Can Do about It* by Joanna L. Robson, DVM. I think it is an excellent explanation of what chiropractic achieves: "There are highways along the body (nerve pathways, meridians). When everything is going well, traffic can get from point A to point B without a hitch. But sometimes there's an accident on the highway and traffic piles up (nerve signals cannot get to the brain or the spinal cord, things don't flow the way they should). As traffic piles up, inflammation occurs because of the blockage. The work in the office doesn't get done (areas in the brain that control the highways begin to shut off because they aren't receiving correct signals). VSMT and acupuncture act like ambulances to restore normal traffic flow by clearing the traffic jams to allow cars to get from point A to point B once again."

In summary, chiropractic works by finding joint subluxations or VSCs—joints that are not moving through their normal range of motion and/or that hurt when you push on them—and then correcting them with an adjustment. The adjustment allows the body to fully correct the VSC and enables the joint to function as it was meant to.

How Does Chiropractic Work on a 1,000-Pound Horse?

When I first considered doing equine chiropractic work, I was concerned I wasn't big or strong enough. Even if I worked out and bulked up a lot of muscle, I'm only 5 feet, 2 inches tall.

But, here's an odd fact: A horse is easier to adjust than a person because of the horse's biomechanical

"Customized" Chiropractic Technique

There are many types of chiropractic techniques used for adjusting. The techniques vary in their focus and methods. Some chiropractors adjust via the bones, others via the ligaments, others use stretching. Some use mechanical aids like activators, drop tables, or foam blocks placed under the individual being adjusted. Each individual chiropractor develops his or her own combination of techniques that work well for them. This becomes his or her "art" and depends on height, size, hand length, and even on personality. (For more on chiropractic techniques, see Eye Spy, p. 24.)

If you've ever been to a chiropractor and it either hurt a lot or didn't help at all, it may be that you needed a different technique. There wouldn't be so many different techniques (over 120!) if they weren't needed.

design. There are several explanations for this, which I describe next.

SUSPENSION BRIDGE STRUCTURE

The horses' biomechanical structure is similar to that of a suspension bridge. This suspension-bridge design

Question~
When is a horse like a suspension bridge?
Answer~
When he's standing up!

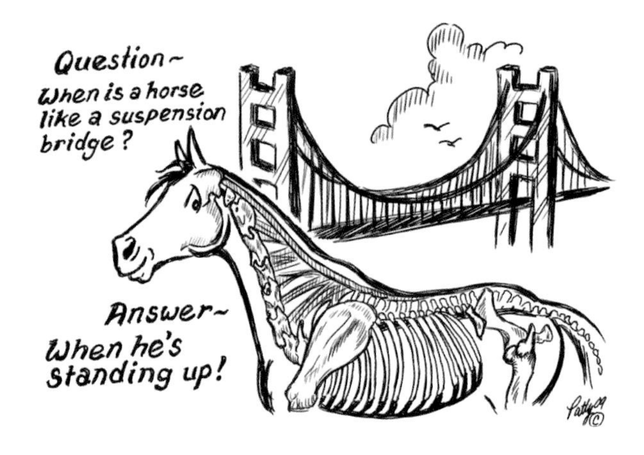

is what allows a thousand pounds or more of horse to stand on top of four comparatively small legs and feet. As you can see in the drawing, the four legs of the horse are the vertical support pillars. The center topline of the horse's back is the main suspension cable. This cable includes the *supraspinatus* ligament, thoracic vertebrae, and dura mater of the spinal cord. The remainder of the horse's barrel (thoracic and abdominal cavities) "hangs" off this cable—via the ribs and barrel muscles—just like the deck of the suspension bridge. Thereby the majority of the horse's weight is transferred, via the suspension cable (topline), over to the vertical support pillars (legs).

When a horse is standing still the only muscle that is activated is the triceps muscle, located above the elbow.

Because the weight is transferred via the "cable" to the legs—completely *unlike* us—*no* muscles are needed to support the horse's standing weight. Only one muscle is in use when the horse is standing still—the triceps muscle, located above the elbow. Because no muscles (other than the triceps) are contracted when the horse is standing still, there are no muscles to "work against" a chiropractic adjustment.

Therefore, it takes much less effort to adjust a horse than it does a human. In humans, a massage is very desirable before an adjustment in order to relax the muscles. This is completely unnecessary in the horse. The muscles are already relaxed. (Note: Any tight muscles in a standing horse indicate that there is something amiss.)

"Come on now," you may scoff. "I can maybe believe this bridge thing about the back, but look at his head. He's got to use his neck muscles to hold up his head!"

Actually, he does not. It takes no muscular effort for the horse to hold his head up. This is because of the *nuchal ligament* on the top of the neck, which is connected to the main "suspension cable" of the back. Rather, it takes muscular effort for the horse to put his head *down*. Therefore, when you notice a horse has tight or contracted muscles standing at rest, even in his neck, this is a good clue that his structure isn't balanced properly.

HORIZONTAL VERTEBRAE

The second major reason that horses are easier to adjust than people is that our back vertebrae are stacked *vertically*—that is, one on top of another. Gravity pulls them down, creating *compressive forces* between each vertebra. When people are adjusted, that compressive force is released (often resulting in a popping or cracking sound). Depending on the amount of muscle involved in the subluxation, the adjustment may take quite a bit of force. I know of several big, muscular guys who need to go to a big, muscular chiropractor to get adjusted!

Now consider the horse's vertebrae: They are lined up horizontally with minimal compressive forces working on them. There are primarily *shear* (sliding) *forces* between horse vertebrae. These shear forces are much less powerful than compressive forces. So even though a horse may weigh 10 times as much as a human, it does not take 10 times the force to adjust him. It actually takes less. Unfortunately, there are uncertified people doing animal chiropractic who don't understand this, and they use hammers and tractors and tranquilizers to get the job done. This is totally unnecessary and can definitely cause harm.

MUSCLE MEMORY

The third advantage horses have over people is due to *muscle memory,* or rather, the lack of it. Whereas a person often needs multiple adjustments because their muscles tend to revert to their previous state, a horse's muscles do not. I used to recheck every horse a week after the first adjustment to look for any subluxations that had returned. Ninety percent of them did not need any adjustments redone and any subluxations that recurred were due to other causes, not muscle memory.

Currently, I'll adjust a horse once, maybe twice at most for the given chiropractic problem. If it returns, most likely there is a *primary problem* more medical in nature causing the subluxation (see When to Consider Chiropractic—and When Not, p. 17). This is a matter for a regular veterinarian to investigate before the *secondary* chiropractic issue can be resolved.

The lack of muscle memory in horses is a good thing! Otherwise we'd be adjusting horses every week. If your horse's chiropractic issue is not at least 90 percent resolved after two treatments (and you followed the prescribed rest and riding recommendations), it's usually time to try something else. That may be a different chiropractor (because as I've mentioned, there are many different techniques), acupuncture, another healing modality, or trying to track down the primary cause with your veterinarian.

HOW OFTEN DOES A HORSE NEED AN ADJUSTMENT?

Horses do not need multiple adjustments to correct their subluxations. However, like any professional athlete, regular chiropractic care is ideal for optimal health and performance.

For example, horses performing at the upper levels of their discipline may need an adjustment every two to three months. Often, however, their owners have them examined for minor chiropractic subluxations once a month and add other modalities like massage or acupuncture, too. One of my clients has a good explanation for this kind of "maintenance": "I keep my horse maintained every month because if you own an expensive, beloved instrument, you need to keep it tuned."

"If you own an expensive, beloved instrument, you need to keep it tuned."

For clients who enjoy pleasure riding on trails, I recommend they have their horses checked every six months to a year—barring any falls, injuries, or illness—and assuming that the list of things able to cause chiropractic subluxations has been addressed (saddle fit, teeth problems, hoof-angle issues, and rider balance, to name just a few). What I find is that once they know how their horse feels when he is correctly aligned, most owners are able to tell when their horse needs an adjustment.

Compensation

A good question that I commonly get asked is, "If it's so easy to adjust horses, why don't they adjust themselves?" The fact is, they *can* adjust themselves. For example, when the horse has a good roll, or when he seeks relief from a pelvic subluxation by leaning his rear end on a bucket in his stall. This is similar to us doing yoga or stretching until one or two of our vertebrae "pop" back into place. You feel a light release of muscles in that area, which can be weird because you probably didn't even notice any tension! Your *not knowing* where there is a problem shows the power of the body's ability to compensate. Here is another example:

When there is only one subluxation, the body is able to reroute the nerve transmissions and clear the area of swelling and inflammation—the process called "compensation." It stops the pain, but it doesn't fix the subluxation.

It's like when you sleep "wrong" and wake up with a stiff neck. The next day it's sore and you wish you could take time off work for a massage. But the following day it's much better. Your pain is gone. But the subluxation is still there. You are able to bend your neck, but not quite as far as you could before—it has a decreased range of motion.

Now when this happens a second time, because the original subluxation is still present, there is even more pain and stiffness. It will take your body longer to reroute the transmissions. But in a week, you'll probably feel fine. Your neck with its decreased range of motion will be in the "minor symptoms" category of the Continuum of Health Chart.

THE CONTINUUM OF HEALTH

- **Optimum Health**
- **Fitness**
- **Wellness**
- **Good Function**
- **No Symptoms (Asymptomatic Dysfunction)**
- **Minor Symptoms**
- **Moderate Symptoms**
- **Severe Symptoms/Disease**
- **Death**

Notice the range of health options in the chart above—from "optimum health" to "no symptoms"—where you could have an issue that you are not aware of because of compensation. Compensation happens in the horse's body as well. In addition, there is redundancy in every system, which means that if some part of the body—say the hock—isn't working quite right, other parts—such as the lumbar section of the back—will "pick up the slack" and there will be no symptoms.

In another example, if part of the horse's circulation system is blocked, the body will enlarge other arteries and veins, and even create new ones to keep the system functioning. By the time you see an "offness," all the compensating systems are overloaded and cannot work at disguising the problem anymore.

A horse does need help with adjustment when he is at the "symptoms stage," that is, when his compensation systems are overloaded and multiple muscles, joints, and ligaments are involved. All these are functionally connected to each other, and the horse needs help unraveling the complexity of the subluxations.

What You Can Do to Help Your Horse

I can tell you that sometimes health and behavior problems are rooted in a chiropractic issue that is pertaining to the horse being out of alignment, and sometimes not. But what I've heard over and over again from caring horse owners is that they wish they had known that chiropractic could fix their horse's problem before:

- Spending thousands of dollars on diagnostics.
- Selling their horse because he couldn't do his job anymore.
- Turning their horse out to pasture for a year.
- Constantly arguing with multiple farriers.
- Buying various training aids.
- Trying new trainers for themselves and/or their horse.
- Thinking for years they just need more lessons or a new saddle.

You get the picture. The good news is that through a series of Body Checkups, you can learn to find exactly where your horse hurts—and whether there is an out-of-alignment issue—before you get stuck in any of the above scenarios. Part Two of this book (see p. 33) contains 27 individual Body Checkups you can perform on the whole horse—from head to tail. By doing these you can discover where, or if, he is subluxated and whether to call your chiropractor.

What I've heard over and over again from caring owners is that they wish they had known that chiropractic could fix their horse's problem before they spent time and money on various wrong "answers."

All the techniques for body checking can be learned by anyone. It just takes patience, a gentle touch—and some practice. Your horse is going to love you and you'll be able to solve many small mysteries before they turn into big problems.

CHAPTER 3

When to Consider Chiropractic—and When Not

Symptoms: What Are They Telling You?

Chiropractic subluxations can be reflected by many different symptoms, whether behavioral, performance-related, or lameness specific. I will deal with all three situations on the pages that follow:

Some horse owners and trainers quickly assume that when horses are resistant they are just being cranky, "mare-ish," stubborn, stupid, lazy, or they just don't want to work. More likely, however, resistance can mean their head, back, legs (or joints), or feet hurt; their saddle doesn't fit; they have no idea what you want; they are being told to do two different things at once; their teeth are hurting their cheeks; their muscles are not in shape for what you're asking; and in the case of a mare, ovulation is making her back sore. And on and on.

Take a look at the sidebar on this page; the lists of potential symptoms can help you "hear" what your horse's behavior is telling you about his discomfort or pain. In addition, be especially mindful when you notice your horse can't manage a movement he used to be able to perform. It might be a sudden change. Maybe there was a known traumatic event—a fall or injury—that caused the problem. However, many times we don't know what happened: The horse just comes in from the pasture and suddenly starts going wide on his third barrel. (And that used to be his best one!) Weird, I know, but it happens a lot.

Common Symptoms that Can Indicate Discomfort or Pain

Behavioral Symptoms

- Crow-hopping, bucking, or rearing
- A "bad attitude," especially when being caught or ridden
- Stable vices such as weaving, stall walking, cribbing
- Not wanting to work
- Leaning on the farrier

Performance Symptoms

- Lack of coordination in gaits
- Lameness that seems to move from limb to limb
- Stiff coming out of stall
- Warming up slowly
- Shying excessively
- Not traveling straight
- Inability to engage hind-quarters

Note: A more detailed, alphabetical list of common symptoms called the Comprehensive Complaints List can be found on page 161. With it, I provide the name of each Body Checkup you need to perform in order to find out whether the symptoms are the result of a chiropractic subluxation of a vertebra or joint, or whether the pain has a different primary cause, more medical in nature (see p. 19).

Or, it might instead be a gradual change (a "worsening") over a few weeks or months. Perhaps the shoulder-in to the left used to be just a bit more difficult than to the right. So you work on it more, but it just keeps getting worse. Months later, even an advanced clinician can't get the shoulder-in to the left.

When your horse is more obviously "off" at a trot rather than a walk, start with your veterinarian.

When your horse is more obviously "off" at a walk, rather than a trot, start with your certified chiropractor.

Even a subtle sign like the horse needing a longer and longer warm-up time can be an indication of underlying pain. Many times we think the horse is just getting older, and in an effort to help we throw in more joint supplements and painkillers. It's time for horse people everywhere to learn if and where their horse is hurting, before taking this (often expensive) step. Everyone will be much happier!

Your horse may show symptoms of lameness. A truly lame horse shows some kind of limp, with or without a head-bob. When I refer to lameness in this book, I am primarily referring to "offness." An offness is when the horse's movement is somehow "wrong" or asymmetrical, but difficult to see or describe. "Offness" can be described in a variety of unique ways. People say things like:

- "He feels like a square peg in a round hole."
- "She feels like two separate horses, front and back, when I ride her."
- "I don't think my horse knows she has a hind end."
- "I can't get him collected at all. He wants to stay on the forehand and trail out his hind end, no matter what."
- "It feels like my horse has stepped in a small hole, but when I look back, there are no holes there."
- "There's just something funky about how he's moving."

When you find yourself saying these types of things it's time to find out where your horse hurts and whether or not the *primary cause* of this problem is something you need to discuss with your veterinarian or chiropractor (for more on *primary causes* see p. 19). First, with offness or lameness, consider this general rule: When your horse is obviously more "off" at *trot rather than walk,* start with your *veterinarian.* When he is obviously more "off" at *walk rather than trot,* start with your *chiropractor.*

For example, if a Western pleasure horse has an obvious head-bob at the trot, and only a very subtle head-bob at the walk, call your veterinarian. Conversely, if a Saddlebred tracks up one inch shorter on the left hind *at the walk,* but tracks up evenly at the trot, it's time to call the chiropractor. This rule is not 100-percent accurate, but it's a great place to start.

A Trainer in the Know

It can be beneficial to work with a trainer familiar with horse chiropractic and experience with the "before and after" of chiropractic treatments. He or she can help you see any offness and discern behavior and performance problems that are happening as a result of pain. Consequently, this type of trainer is worth any additional fees up front because potentially, he or she can save you a lot of money in vet bills later. (A list of horse professionals that have passed a proficiency exam covering the entire chiropractic Body Checkups program is available at www.wheredoesmyhorsehurt.com.)

Primary Causes: When Chiropractic Is Not the Answer

The behavior, performance, and "offness" symptoms we just discussed are typical of horses with chiropractic subluxations that need correcting. Sometimes, however, horses can have these same symptoms, yet the cause may not necessarily be chiropractic. The main, or *primary,* cause of the problem is what needs to be addressed first.

Primary causes are many: saddle fit; vitamin and mineral imbalance; hoof angles; teeth issues; leg-joint arthritis; tendon or muscle overstrain; medical internal issues; and even a rider who needs chiropractic adjustment.

SADDLE FIT

Saddle fit is an extremely important issue, as most horses' saddles do *not* fit. Horses do much better when their saddle does not cause them pain or discomfort. It only takes a small pressure point the size of a dime to cause a subluxation. Fitting a saddle correctly can be tricky, but with a little study you can learn how to do it. I highly recommend Dr. Joyce Harman's books and DVDs on fitting both English and Western saddles (www.horseandriderbooks.com).

VITAMIN AND MINERAL SUPPLEMENTS

Why does nutrition matter? It may seem strange that overall poor nutrition caused by a lack of necessary vitamins and supplements factors into a horse becoming subluxated, but it does happen. Perhaps I should say that inadequate nutrition certainly doesn't contribute to the horse's body being able to stay in alignment.

A horse's vitamin and mineral needs fluctuate along with any changes made in his hay or grain consumption; his work levels; weather temperatures and barometric pressures; and vaccinations, to name just a few items. In addition, lack of one specific mineral can cause others to become unbalanced. For example, when a horse is low in mineral A, mineral B becomes too *high* and high levels of mineral B cause minerals C and D to become *low.* This unbalancing effect continues until the horse's entire system becomes completely out of whack.

NOT every behavioral problem, performance issue, and lameness can be fixed with chiropractic treatments.

Does a horse look sick when he is deficient in one mineral? Unlikely. But he'll eventually become desperate to get that mineral: He'll chew wood, eat dirt, or, if in the wild, travel for miles and miles to find the one weed needed for balance.

When a horse's system is unbalanced it will affect him in different ways, depending on which minerals

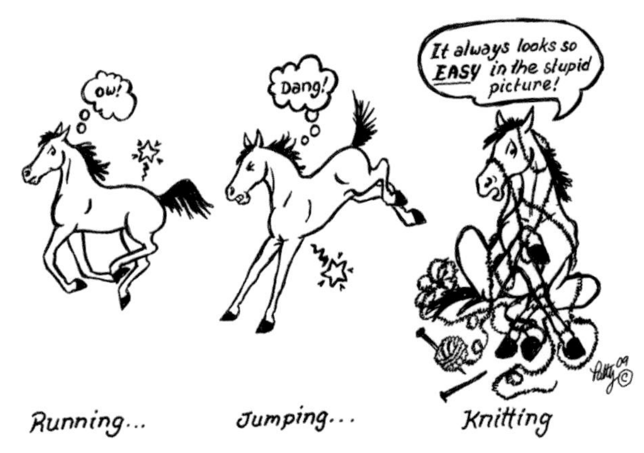

are involved. Let's say that the imbalance causes his muscles and ligaments to become too "tight." Should the horse stumble, his body is not flexible enough to allow him to recover his balance.

Obviously a fall will cause subluxations, but even if the horse manages to "save" himself and doesn't actually fall, the "pulling" on his inflexible muscles will cause subluxations, anyway. And, when vitamin or mineral imbalance is significant, heavy work alone may be enough to cause subluxations. This is why it is really important to offer the correct vitamins and minerals at all times.

When to Supplement

There are some clues as to when it is a good idea to add supplements to your horse's diet. First, your horse's hair coat and hooves should be healthy. If not, there is most likely a vitamin or mineral deficiency. A shiny coat is healthy; dull hair or dry flaky skin is not. Hooves should not have cracks or wavy lines on them. If your horse goes barefoot, his hooves should not chip off excessively.

Second, some horses show signs of needing a vitamin or mineral by eating dirt or sand; eating bark or weeds that other horses will not; licking wood or metal; licking you incessantly; or drinking mud puddles. A lot of people believe these behaviors to be a "cute" habit—some horses have had them, even since birth—but they should be taken seriously and, if possible, the reason for them tracked down. When a horse is severely deficient in a vitamin or mineral (or the opposite—has way too much), there will be specific signs of illness. These symptoms are too numerous to list and you should involve your veterinarian at this point.

Third, you can check for vitamin and mineral needs with a hair mineral analysis. Even though you may be giving the correct amounts of vitamins and minerals, your horse may not be absorbing the correct amounts and hair analysis is a good way of finding out.

Send some of your horse's mane (usually with the root) to a lab that does this kind of work. (You can do a Web search for "horse hair mineral analysis" or your veterinarian may have a recommendation.) Costs vary but typically range from $50 to $150. It is worth doing, if for no other reason than making sure that you are not wasting supplements!

Free-Choice Supplementation

You may well ask if correcting such a dietary imbalance will take months to solve the behavior or lameness issue. Surprisingly, it won't. When you offer *separate, free-choice* (not in the horse's feed) vitamins and minerals, your horse's system can become balanced in three to eight weeks. Just don't be surprised if your horse wants to eat 20 pounds of a certain mineral! (Don't worry, horses are quite capable of balancing themselves—as long as they are not sick or debilitated.)

You can purchase separate vitamins and minerals of all kinds. However, vitamin E and selenium are always distributed together (see more on this on p. 21), as are calcium and phosphorus, because they balance each other out. Calcium and phosphorus also come in different ratios, depending whether your horse is still growing or not. But—before you think this is too complicated—all you need to do is *offer* them to your horse, and he will eat exactly the amount he needs. I also recommend feeding minerals separately from salt. The reason for this is that once a horse has enough salt, he will no longer eat a mineral mix that includes salt, even though he may still be mineral deficient.

Selenium

Consult your veterinarian (or local agricultural extension office) for the types and amount of supplements recommended for your area due to its soil. Take selenium for example. In certain areas of the United States, selenium deficiency is a problem. In other areas, there is an excess of selenium in the soil. Selenium is necessary for healthy muscles that can completely contract, relax, and stretch. A selenium-deficient horse's muscles feel tight all the time, and his movement is stiff.

Psyllium

Not to be confused with selenium, psyllium (marketed as Sand Clear and Equi Aid®) is a plant that clears the horse's intestines of sand or dirt picked up by eating off the ground; consuming it in hay or feed; or from just plain old liking to eat sand and dirt. You don't have to live in a desert to find sand in your horse's gut, which can be recognized when a horse looks bloated. Many a case of "ADR" (Ain't Doin' Right) has been cured by giving the horse psyllium, so I suggest using it as recommended by your veterinarian.

FEET

Incorrect hoof angles, under-run heels, and contracted heels are just a few of the many problems commonly seen in the horse's feet. The horse's body compensates for these, and this compensating eventually causes subluxations. For example, when a horse has one low heel, that leg is nearer to the ground. For the horse's body to stay level on the other three legs, his shoulder angle has to open up with the top of the shoulder blade actually moving higher than its normal position. This puts an uneven pressure across the withers and they become subluxated.

Be sure that your horse's feet are in good shape. Ask your veterinarian or farrier if you're not sure what good feet look like.

TEETH

Be sure your horse's teeth are floated by a competent dentist. A hook (or hooks), or other dental issues can cause a horse to "freeze" his jaw (i.e. clamp his teeth together) to avoid pain. You will not be able to see him doing this but the action causes a lack of flexion in the poll, which therefore promotes stiffness—and eventually subluxations—all the way down the back.

There is a range of competence in dentistry. There are good dentists, bad dentists, and everything in between. Just because someone is a veterinarian or is a dentist that has "learned with the best" does not necessarily make them competent. Ask around.

ARTHRITIS

The same kind of compensatory situation can happen with arthritis. When the right hock is arthritic, the left sacroiliac and lumbar joints will be subluxated. This is simply because they are being overused due to their compensating for the right hock. In this situation, the primary cause of arthritis needs to be addressed before the chiropractic subluxations can be permanently corrected.

TENDON OR LIGAMENT OVERUSE

Let's say that your horse is overusing his right suspensory ligament. Regardless of the reason—chiropractic or otherwise—in order to protect it, he will compensate and subtly shift some weight over to the left leg. Because the horse's legs work in a diagonal manner, the right hind leg will also have to compensate, and he'll probably have a subluxated right sacroiliac joint. So, yes, there is a chiropractic subluxation, however, the primary cause is the right suspensory ligament. This ligament must be healed first. Then the secondary chiropractic subluxations can be corrected through adjustment.

Multiple visits to correct the exact same chiropractic pattern are not the answer.

MEDICAL ISSUES

If you suspect a medical issue is causing your horse's behavior, performance, or lameness symptoms, obviously your veterinarian should be involved. A good example is ulcers, which are very common. Horses with them may appear "on edge" unable to concentrate or learn new things, or to keep still. However, there are many horses with ulcers and no obvious symptoms. Ask your veterinarian to look your horse over if you see any suspicious behavior or if your horse's chiropractic adjustments do not "hold."

A RIDER IN NEED OF CHIROPRACTIC ADJUSTMENT

Believe it or not, out-of-alignment riders can cause their horse to be in need of adjustment. For example, a rider whose pelvis is crooked (one hip looks higher than the other and her stirrups feel uneven) distributes her weight unevenly across the saddle. This causes subluxations in the thoracic vertebrae and ribs of the horse.

Chiropractor or Veterinarian?

It is challenging to figure out whether symptoms of discomfort are from chiropractic subluxations or other primary causes that need a veterinarian's attention, and which professional to aim for, at first. I will discuss these options case by case in the 27 Body Checkups (see Part Two, p. 33).

Sometimes, you can start with a chiropractor but find the problem keeps coming back. In another case, there is a prior injury (for example, a tendon laceration that has built up scar tissue) that repeatedly causes chiropractic subluxations. A chiropractic maintenance schedule is certainly reasonable; however, multiple visits to correct the exact same chiropractic pattern are not the answer. Be wary of a chiropractor who tells you that due to muscle memory, multiple visits are needed for an adjustment to fully hold. When you continue to have the same problem over and over again, it's time to search for a different primary cause.

In summary, when you have a behavioral, performance, or offness problem with your horse, first, be sure your horse's teeth, feet, diet, and saddle fit are all in good shape. Then call your vet when you have an offness that is more obvious at the trot. Otherwise, call your certified chiropractor for consultation.

CHAPTER 4

How to Find a Good Chiropractor

In your search for a good equine chiropractor, I first recommend you educate yourself about the laws regarding animal chiropractic in your state. Typically, a state's veterinary medical board will have this information, though sometimes you may also need to contact the human chiropractic board. The best way to find this is through an Internet search.

In most states there are one of two laws, or some version of them: 1) The animal chiropractor must be a veterinarian; or 2) The animal chiropractor must be "under the supervision" of a veterinarian. "Under the supervision" does not mean that the veterinarian has to be there, but rather that he is familiar with the horse and has referred the owner to the chiropractor.

You need to find a certified chiropractor, and ideally one who is practicing legally. Remember, such a person can be either a veterinarian (DVM) or a chiropractor (DC) to become certified in animal chiropractic. However, some state laws may require only veterinarians do chiropractic work on animals. I do know some people who try to adjust animals that do so because there is no one else available in their area. They're either self-taught or have "tagged along" with another animal chiropractor for a while. They mean well. But, still, it's a sticky situation for them to be in. Some do a decent job; but some are harmful to the animals. These people typically have no paperwork or even a receipt for you. (If there were paperwork, the state boards would have the needed evidence to stop them from working.) Without a written record, it makes it hard for you to keep track of what is happening with your horse's chiropractic issues. What is very best for your horse is to have your veterinarian—or certified chiropractor working with a vet (if that's legal in your state)—do your chiropractic work. Having both the veterinary knowledge and the chiropractic training is ideal.

A Sad Story

Once I met a farrier who was "adjusting horses" on the side for an added $25 on top of his shoeing fee. He asked me if I thought he could have made a horse lame while doing a shoulder adjustment. He described his technique, which included a lot of pulling, wrenching, and "throwing" of the shoulder.

The horse was now unable to move his leg forward, although he could still fully bear weight on that leg. From the farrier's description, it was most likely that the horse had radial nerve paralysis, and yes, he caused that. Sadly, the owner was now stuck with a completely lame horse that may, or may not ever get better.

Chiropractic Associations

When searching for a chiropractor, start with the American Veterinary Chiropractic Association (www.animalchiropractic.org). This organization certifies both veterinarians and human chiropractors for animal chiropractic care. Its Web site lists many of the available certified veterinarians and chiropractors by state, and includes links. Not all certified practitioners are listed on the AVCA Web site, for various reasons; you can call the AVCA office and ask directly about an individual and find out whether he or she has been through the course modules, and passed the examination (see p. 4 where I discussed chiropractic education).

When a veterinarian or chiropractor is certified with the AVCA, he or she may choose to add the initials "CAC" to a business card. This stands for Certified in Animal Chiropractic.

In the UK, visit the McTimoney Chiropractic Association (MCA) Web site (www.mctimoneychiropractic.org). MCA is the only chiropractic association in the UK to have a specific group of chiropractors qualified and trained to treat animals. MCA has its own college in Oxfordshire that offers a two year post-graduate course in chiropractic for animals.

All these certifications and degrees can be confusing and people come with all sorts of different backgrounds. Usually they like to tell you their story, so just ask about their background and credentials. If they get upset and act offended, treat it as a red flag and find someone different.

I do realize, however, that there is a shortage of legal, certified practitioners. Most equine veterinarians are far too busy to get the extra certification needed for chiropractic, let alone have the time to add another service to their practice. As this is unfortunately the case, here are few more ideas for how to find a, qualified practitioner.

Ask Your Veterinarian

Veterinarians often see the "before and after" of a horse's condition, which is why they are in a good position to evaluate chiropractic care. They are also familiar with animal chiropractors in their area. There is a caveat, however. A veterinarian who refers a client to a person who is practicing chiropractic without a license may himself be held liable if anything goes wrong. For this reason, some veterinarians will not recommend someone unless that person is a legally practicing, certified animal chiropractor. Explain to your vet that you just want an opinion, not necessarily a referral, and you should get a lot more information regarding chiropractors in your region.

Eye Spy

Whether or not you can get good referrals, watching an animal chiropractor work is one of the best ways to see if a person is doing a good job. Call a prospective practitioner and request information on his education, experience, and references, and then ask if you can watch him work on a horse.

Look for two things: the horse's response and what the chiropractor is doing.

WATCH THE HORSE'S REACTION

First, if the horse doesn't like the animal chiropractor, go with his instinct. Horses do not mind being around most people so when you see a horse reacting poorly to even the presence of an individual, don't ignore it. Horses can also sense whether or not you are trying to care for them.

If the horse initially likes the chiropractor, watch his expression during the adjustment. Signs of too much force include: laying ears flat back, trying to bite, and kicking out. Some adjustments can be a bit uncomfortable because of the need to put pressure on a body part that already hurts. However, it is only for a second or two. It's like having a bad bruise pressed on momentarily as a warm cloth is added: You flinch but then relax when you feel the pleasant warmth.

So, it's okay when you see brief tension followed by relaxation after the adjustment. You may also see signs of endorphin release from the adjustment. These signs include: licking of the lips; chewing; passing gas; lowering the head; and looking sleepy or glassy-eyed. Not all horses show these signs of endorphin release, particularly when it is their first session of any type of bodywork. But you are just looking for the horse being comfortable overall.

OBSERVE THE CHIROPRACTOR'S TECHNIQUES

Force

Remember that there are many different chiropractic techniques (see p. 11). You want to be sure that the chiropractor understands that the horse does not need a tremendous amount of force for an adjustment.

Some examples of too much force include: the horse being tied to anything to "help" the adjustment, such as a trailer or the barn wall; the horse being laid on the ground (with or without tranquilizers); hammers or mallets being used more forcefully than a light tapping; or the horse's leg or other body part being strongly jerked. Anything being done that makes you gasp or your eyes widen is being done too forcefully.

Activator

An "activator" is used by some human chiropractors as an adjustment tool. It's made of metal and it contains an extremely fast moving internal piece. This internal piece is the part that is doing the adjusting. You hear a lot of clicking sounds when it is used. This tool works very well on people.

The theory behind the use of this tool is physics. The physics equation referenced in force chiropractic is: Force = Mass x Acceleration. The force is equal to the mass multiplied by the acceleration of the mass. So, for example, a large man can punch very slowly and knock his opponent out. However, a smaller guy (smaller mass) can move his arm at lightning speed (faster acceleration) and also

Any technique being used that makes you gasp or your eyes widen is too forceful.

Questions to Ask a Prospective Chiropractor

- Which veterinarians do you work with or who are you supervised by?
- Do you have references?
- Will you explain what is happening as you work?
- What are your aftercare instructions?
- Will you provide a record of adjustments and a payment receipt?
- Can I call you later if I have any questions?

knock his opponent out. Activators are designed so that their very low mass is made up for by the extreme speed of the interior piece.

Activators do adjust vertebrae, though not, as is often incorrectly thought, by forcing a bone back into place. To quote Dr. Joanna Robson again (see p. 11) "...it is the effect of a quick motion that causes a reflexive relaxation of the muscles surrounding the joint and allows the body's innate intelligence to return it to balance."

An activator in use.

However, I have not found this tool to work well on all areas of the horse. I believe one reason it doesn't is because of the amount of muscle the activator needs to work through.

Regardless, an activator won't hurt a horse. A word of warning: When you have a new chiropractor and he uses this tool, make sure he actually touches the horse with his hands, too. I've heard stories of chiropractors who have taken only 10 minutes to "click all over" a horse, "adjusting" everything, and then charging the owner $150! It's one of the reasons why chiropractic has been viewed with skepticism in some quarters.

Time and Extent

A horse cannot receive a proper adjustment in a 10-minute session. I'm referring to a first-time adjustment, not a recheck or a horse that has had regular adjustments prior to the one you are witnessing. I can do a first-time adjustment in 30 minutes, if I don't pause to explain anything to the owner. However, it is my preference to talk as I go and answer questions, so I usually take 45 minutes to an hour.

I do know good chiropractors where speed is one of their primary goals. They can adjust a horse in 20 to 25 minutes. However, what is important is

The Horse Always Knows

My "non-horsey" friends used to always ask me if I was scared when I performed veterinary work. They asked because they thought it likely that horses would either run away or try to hurt me if I had to give them a vaccine or tranquilizer shot. I explained that I've always found that horses "know" when you're trying to help. They don't run away. They stand still and look you in the eye to see what you mean to do. This is actually taught at chiropractic certification school. The instructors say, "Horses know your intent. Be sure you're doing this for the right reasons." This is in reference to those who get into the animal chiropractic business only for money—without caring for the animal at all. In my opinion, there are very few people doing animal chiropractic that don't care about the animals. But there are some. So my point is, watch the horse's response. He knows!

that you see the chiropractor check every part listed in the Body Checkups in this book, and if not, ask why he or she hasn't! (By the way, the Body Checkups I describe in Part Two of this book are the most straightforward ones I know and the ones I use every day. However, there are many ways of checking horses. You want to be certain the chiropractor you are watching checks every part of the body, whichever technique or method he is using.)

A PROPER ADJUSTMENT

As just discussed, by a "proper adjustment" I mean you should see the chiropractor check every possible part of the horse including: the atlas, occiput, neck, C7, sternum, withers, thoracic, lumbar, sacrum, sacroiliac, all the leg joints, and the ribs (see more about this starting on p. 33). Many chiropractors don't check ribs because they think the ribs will align themselves after the other major parts have been adjusted. I have not found this to be true. The ribs are extremely important to adjust, primarily because the saddle sits directly above them.

Also, make sure the chiropractor actually adjusts all body parts that need it. Some like to return and adjust in stages. This is unnecessary—unless, of course, the horse is trying to "kill" him. Then it's necessary—for the chiropractor!

A good chiropractor will tell you when your problem cannot be treated successfully with chiropractic adjustment, and should instead be dealt with by your veterinarian. For example, if I find that a horse's atlas is difficult to adjust, then I ask about his dental history, check the teeth, and refer the owner to her veterinarian for a teeth float, if needed. As mentioned earlier, uneven teeth, or teeth "hooks" in the back of the mouth, cause the atlas to repeatedly become subluxated.

AFTERCARE INSTRUCTIONS

Lastly, exercise and work routines must be altered after adjustments are made. Generally speaking, horses need a few days off with no riding and plenty of turnout where they can walk around comfortably. There are still some chiropractors around who were certified long ago when a week of stall rest was recommended. This has been found to be

A good chiropractor will tell you when your problem cannot be treated with chiropractic adjustment and you need to contact your vet, instead.

The Importance of Checking Every Body Part

I started working on Gabby, a seven-year-old Andalusian mare who was doing Second Level dressage work, when she had been stuck at that level for a few years because she couldn't do flying changes. Gabby had previously been adjusted every month for a couple of years by another chiropractor who used the 10-minute "clicker" (activator) method I described on p. 26.

When I started checking Gabby's ribs, her owner asked what I was doing; she didn't even realize that a horse's ribs should be checked. It turned out that the majority of the mare's ribs were subluxated. It was actually difficult to tell that they were subluxated because of the mare's extremely high pain tolerance (common in Andalusians). But I noticed that she stopped breathing and "braced" her rib cage whenever I attempted to check that area. (Note: This may be the only sign shown by pain-tolerant horses.) After she was adjusted—including her ribs—she performed flying changes with ease.

unnecessary—and possibly detrimental. The biomechanical structure of the horse is what enables adjustments to stay in place, and walking around helps the neural proprioceptive reset.

The chiropractor should suggest a "check in" phone call if the owner notices residual soreness for longer than five days. Any horse may be muscle-sore for one or two days after an adjustment, but more than five days of dragging around and not feeling good is too long. On a couple of occasions I have had owners call me because their horse was still muscle-sore and moping around after two weeks. In both cases, it was discovered the horse had a preexisting liver condition unbeknownst to the owner.

A "Good Chiropractic Session" in a Nutshell

Force Used	• Low force preferable • NO excessive force
Horse's Reaction	• Likes chiropractor • Comfortable overall (except very brief, minor discomfort from the adjustment thrust for some types of treatment) • Shows endorphin-release signs (not mandatory)
Length of Session	• 20 minutes minimum to 60 minutes maximum (not counting breaks)
Extent of Checkup	• Covers all Body Checkups outlined in this book (see Part Two, p. 33) • Provides aftercare instructions • Invites post-session phone calls with questions/concerns

CHAPTER 5

Body Checkup Fundamentals

Before you get to actually performing the 27 Body Checkups I provide in this book on your horse, you need to read this chapter. Why? Because the devil is in the details. Not literally, of course: The devil is the one causing your horse to have problems! But educating yourself thoroughly about the practicalities and learning by example will make performing Body Checkups easier for you—and for your horse.

What Are Body Checkups?

The 27 Body Checkups I describe in this book are step-by-step descriptions of how to check various parts of your horse's body for pain, discomfort, limited range of movement, and other signs that he may be suffering from a subluxation (and thus benefit from a chiropractic session). Body Checkups *do not* adjust the horse or otherwise enable you to correct a problem—they simply help you identify the whereabouts and probable cause of, for example, a lameness you are noticing, or bring to your attention an issue with joints or bones that may still be without symptoms (giving you an opportunity to "nip" a problem in the bud). This way, you can avoid repeat diagnostic attempts (that can become very expensive); limit the occurrence of "mystery lameness"; and keep your horse free of pain and his movement optimal. Body Checkups tell you whether and when to call a veterinarian, chiropractor, horse dentist, saddle-fitting expert, or farrier, or perhaps how to better manage vitamin and supplement intake (see p. 19 for more about "primary causes").

Hand Positions

Sometimes, I recommend you use a specific part of your hand for a Body Checkup, such as the side edge or the thumb base, but if you find a better way for you—go for it!

When a Body Checkup calls for the use of your fingers, use the *pads* of your fingers, not the tips. Avoid using "pokey fingers." By "pokey," I don't mean slow. I mean "poke-y," as if someone is poking you in the side. Irritating. Hurtful.

A few areas that I reference in Part Two (p. 33) include: the side edge of the hand, the pisiform area, and the thumb base. I also provide specific hand positions for checking the horse's ribs (see photos of these areas and positions on p. 30).

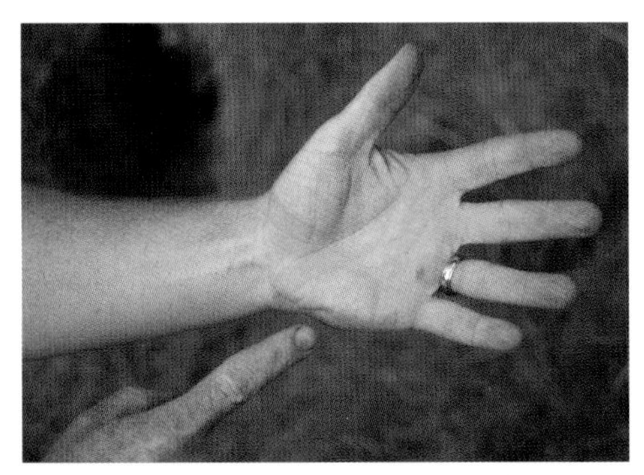

The side edge of the hand.

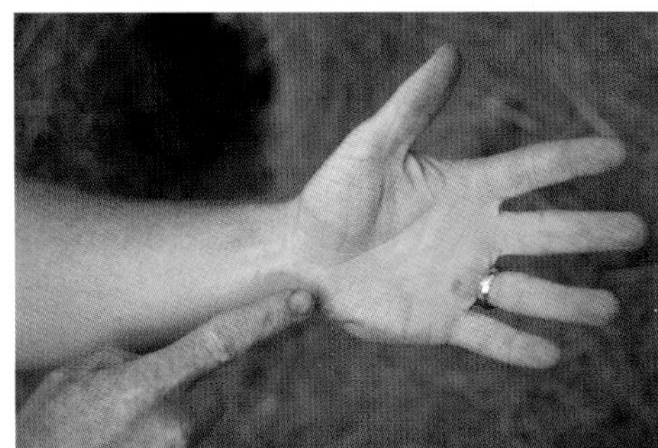

The pisiform area.

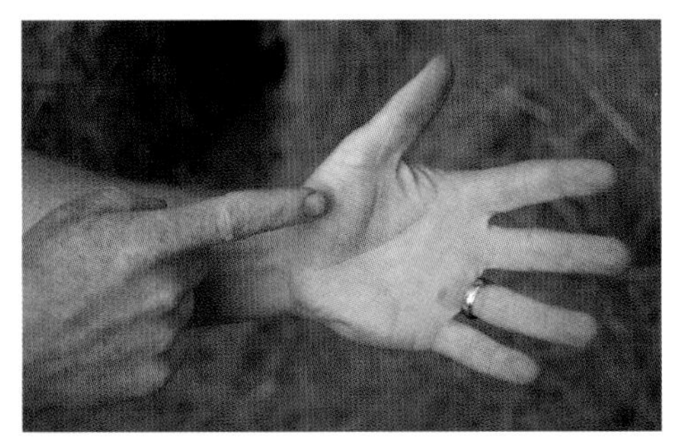

The thumb base.

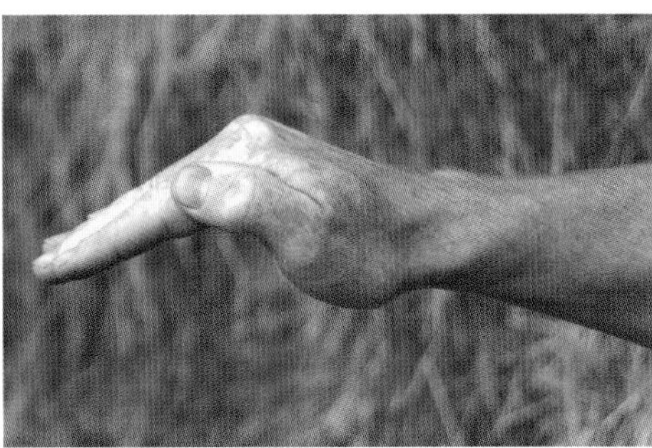

The specific hand position for checking the ribs (p. 117).

Time, Pressure, and Patience

Just like any other horse skill, learning to do Body Checkups takes practice, which can seem slow at first. As a professional, I can do all of them in less than five minutes, but I remember when it took me 10 minutes just to do the Sacroiliac Joint Checkup (p. 134)!

If you commit to doing all 27 Body Checkups every day for three weeks, I believe you can then reduce the length of time it takes to an overall 5 to 10 minutes. And, then you can just check your horse once a week, or as needed.

When you begin, give yourself lots of time. Be patient with yourself. Be patient with your horse—he may think you've gone crazy! It may take him a few times to realize that, yes, you do want his leg to wiggle like that.

As you get familiar with your horse's body, also try checking him before and after exercise. It's useful to know the difference between "cold" and warmed-up muscles, tendons, and ligaments—especially when your horse has an issue that you can only feel when riding him.

Try to do these Body Checkups on many different horses. Just as riding other people's horses improves your ability to ride your own, so will doing Body Checkups on different animals help you more accurately diagnose the location of your own horse's pain and discomfort. Comparing the variations in different horses' range of motion is invaluable.

PRESSURE

As you practice the Checkups, use the lightest hand (or finger) pressure necessary. There are two reasons for this. First, the horse will appreciate the light pressure, particularly in sore areas, and will respond well to lightness once he realizes what you want. Second, it is actually easier to feel your horse's body when you use a light pressure because the "feelers" in your fingertips become deadened the more pressure you put on them.

So when I say in the pages ahead to use "light pressure" or "gently move," it is intended to keep your ability to feel with your hands and fingertips available. "Light" is approximately the "weight" you would use to check a peach for ripeness. If you see the skin color under the tip of your fingernails become white, you are using way too much pressure. Try it now by pushing on your forearm to see how much pressure causes your fingers to lose circulation and the skin underneath your fingernails to turn white.

Stoic (pain-tolerant) horses do need more pressure in order for you to see a response. However, *always* start *lightly* and slowly press harder, but only when necessary. How do you know if more pressure is needed? This mostly comes with practice. It can help to notice other clues that show you the horse may be "hiding" painful areas, such as if the horse:

- Holds his breath
- Becomes very still
- Gets very "busy" (dancing around, shaking his head, trying to leave)

Sensitivity, Response, and Range of Motion

There is quite a difference between different horses' *sensitivity* and *response* to touch and pressure—from a skin twitch to stomping feet.

I'm only talking about a horse's response to Body Checkups, not the way he acts generally: A horse may be very sensitive to a Checkup, but "dull" at other times—or, vice versa. For example, when doing the Rib Checkup on a Thoroughbred, you barely have to press down on a subluxated rib to get a big response (skin twitching, ears back, and the "evil-eye"). However, a Warmblood with the same type of rib subluxation may require you press down so hard that you strain your wrists, and even then, you may only get a tiny muscle twitch in response.

"Light" pressure is approximately the pressure used to check a peach for ripeness.

The *range of motion* of different horses' joints varies considerably, also.

Differences in horses' sensitivity, response, and joint range of motion are caused by a number of factors including: age, breed, use, gender, muscle soreness, and even the horse's familiarity with bodywork.

Age Younger horses are more sensitive, have greater (and quicker) responses, and have close to perfect range of motion.

Breed Breed is the most important factor when it comes to sensitivity and responsiveness. Hot-blooded breeds, such as Thoroughbreds and Arabians, are more sensitive and respond accordingly, while Warmbloods, such as Hanoverians, and often Quarter Horses, are much less sensitive and responsive, in general. Cold bloods like Belgians and Percherons, (draft types) are actually more sensitive but less responsive than most Warmbloods. In addition, draft horses have a larger range of motion in their joints than you might expect.

Use By "use" I'm not referring to a type of riding discipline, but rather amount of use. A horse "lightly used" for 10 years will have more sensitivity, responsiveness, and range of motion than a horse that has been used "hard" from an early age. Because of variations in use, you can have two seven-year-olds, one with perfect range of motion in all joints and the other with vastly decreased motion. A horse that has been ridden hard has learned to "toughen up," and his sensitivity and response mechanisms have been dulled.

Gender Typically mares have a greater sensitivity and response than geldings, particularly when they're in season. Stallions often show greater sensitivity but a more restrained response than geldings. Range of motion is unaffected by gender.

Familiarity with Bodywork The more "good bodywork" a horse has received, the greater his sensitivity and response will be. By good bodywork, I mean that the horse enjoyed the session and the work had a helpful effect. But, when he has had an unpleasant or painful bodywork experience, his reaction to the next bodywork session may increase, resulting in his acting up. He may dance around or even try to kick because he wants it to stop. However, if he has been punished for this type of active reaction to bodywork in the past, his response may instead decrease: His brain blocks the pain and he "shrinks inside himself."

A horse's range of motion may also be increased as a result of good bodywork.

You Can Do This!

You may well be feeling after reading about all these variations and complications, as well as all the sensitivity stuff, that it is going to be way too difficult to tell where your horse hurts. It's not! You can do it! I have given seminars to all manner of people, from a trainer with 30 years' horse experience, to a grandmother who brought her 11-year-old granddaughter to ride at the barn where I was working that day. And, they all "got" this! Some people may learn a bit faster than others. But if you go at your own pace, you will learn to tell where your horse hurts—maybe even before your horse shows any signs of hurting!

PART TWO

27 Body Checkups You Can Do on Your Horse

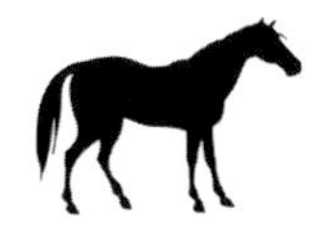

Chiropractic Body Checkups

How To

Where Does My Horse Hurt does not teach you how to adjust horses; it teaches you how to tell *if* your horse hurts, where your horse hurts, and whether you have a chiropractic issue. It also gives you some ideas of what else could be causing the behavior, performance issue, or lameness or "offness," thus providing you important information so you can be the one to help your horse stop hurting.

Step One

Review the Top 10 Complaints List

In no particular order the most common issues I've seen during my career as a veterinarian and a chiropractor are listed in the chart at the right.

Because these issues are so common, I've created quick-reference flow charts to help those dealing with them to formulate a plan of action and follow it. You can find one for each of the above complaints in the Appendix on pp. 155–160. When your horse's problem is on this list, simply follow the handy Problem-Solving Flow Chart provided that tells you which Body Checkups you should do to diagnose the cause of your horse's problem. (When your horse's problem is not on this list, proceed to Step Two.) After you have located the appropriate Problem-Solving Flow Chart, go on to Step Three.

TOP 10 COMPLAINTS	
1	Short-striding (or off) in front
2	Short-striding (or off) behind
3	Head-shy or ear-shy
4	Difficulty picking up, maintaining, or changing leads
5	Difficulty with collection or impulsion
6	Difficulty with bending
7	"Girthy"
8	Travels wide and/or drops shoulder on turns
9	Rider feels crooked or saddle slips to one side
10	Horse feels stiff or is cold-backed

Step Two
Review the Comprehensive Complaints List

When your horse's problem is not one of those described in the Top 10 Complaints List, review the alphabetical Comprehensive Complaints List in the Appendix (p. 161). There, you'll see that next to each complaint are the Body Checkups you need to perform in order to find out if your horse has any chiropractic subluxations.

Step Three
Do Each Suggested Body Checkup

You can do Body Checkups in any order. I personally find it best to do them beginning at the head and working toward the tail, so this is the way I present them to you, starting on page 43. When done in a sensible order, it is less likely that you'll accidentally skip one.

However, as an alternative you can do the Checkups by their degree of difficulty. I have laid out what I call the "Challenge-Level Method" for those who prefer, for example, to do the easiest ones first. I have allotted each Body Checkup a number of "stars" (☆), from one star (the easiest) to four (the most difficult). It should be noted that while five-star Checkups exist (see sidebar, p. 38), they are beyond the scope of this book. If you feel that your horse may have a problem with a five-star Checkup area, please call your certified chiropractor.

Step Four
Review Diagnoses

Typically, you will find you've had to do at least five Body Checkups. Review these Checkups' diagnoses and make an initial plan. The number of probable subluxations discovered determines your next move:

1) Three or fewer probable subluxations indicate the horse's issue is unlikely to be from a primary chiropractic origin. Yes, the horse may well have some areas that need to be resolved via chiropractic, but they are probably as a result of his body compensating for his primary problem—this is a general rule, not hard fact. Note that in the summary at the end of each Checkup, I've included a list of possible primary problems to explore.

2) More than three subluxations and you most likely are dealing with a chiropractic issue. Now it's time to for you to call a certified chiropractor to perform an adjustment—or more than one.

Step Five
Recheck the Horse's Symptoms

Once you have had your horse adjusted, give it a few days (depending on your chiropractor's recommendation) and recheck his symptoms. If they still exist, start over with the Body Checkups and consider going over all of them with your chiropractor to get his input.

Three Sample Checkups

Example One

Chiropractic Adjustment Works

Let's say you have a lovely, five-year-old, bay mare (I'll call her Regina), and she is consistently tripping. She trips enough that you've already had your veterinarian to look at her, but, needless to say, the day he came she did not trip the entire hour he observed her! Now, with this book in hand, you are armed with information and ready to try again to help solve Regina's problem.

Step One: First, you check the Top Ten Complaints List on p. 35. You find that tripping is not on it, so you continue on to Step Two.

Step Two: You look through the Comprehensive Complaints List (p. 161), and while doing so, you are reminded of a few more symptoms that Regina has displayed from time to time. You write down all her symptoms, and make a list of the Body Checkups you need to do.

Regina's Symptoms

- Tripping
- Short striding
- Sometimes "off" in front

Regina's Body Checkups: To Do

C7, p. 60; Shoulder Blade, p. 66; Shoulder, p.69; Elbow, p. 77; Knee, p. 81; Splint Bone, p. 87; Fetlock, p. 90; Sesamoid Bones, p. 94; Pastern, p. 98; Coffin Joint, p. 102; Withers, p. 108; Ribs, p. 117

You start thinking, "Yikes, that is sooo many! I can't learn all of these Checkups!" But you take a deep breath and just start through the step-by-step instructions, looking for subluxations. What happens next is interesting: You can't find anything wrong with the shoulder blade or knee, but the C7, the shoulder, and the elbow all seem to be subluxated.

You think one splint bone is also possibly subluxated but aren't quite certain. However, now you don't have to finish all the exams! You already have found more than three probable subluxations, so you know that you need to get a certified chiropractor to look at your horse.

Your chiropractor comes out, adjusts Regina, who becomes immediately much happier with a bright look in her eye. After a few days rest, you take her out for light exercise and she is not tripping and her stride is definitely improved! But, you remember that the problems seem to be present some days but not others. So you continue to watch her for the next few days. After a week of no symptoms, you finally start celebrating! You were the one to solve your horse's mystery. Yes, the chiropractor did the physical work, but you took the initiative to find out where Regina hurt and how you could help her. Congratulations!

Example Two

An Adjustment Is Not the Whole Solution

After your sweet success with Regina, you are not overwhelmed when your daughter's pony, Pumpkin, starts acting up. Pumpkin, who has always been "Queen of the Ponies" (and all horses, as well), suddenly is not listening to your daughter. They had been jumping up to 2 feet and looking as cute as a

Challenge Level Method

If you are a bodyworker, or are simply interested in the finer details of the Body Checkups, I have developed a method of doing them that I call the Challenge Level Method. It is not mandatory.

Each Checkup has been given a star designation (see Chart 1). One star ☆ is the easiest Checkup to do and four stars ☆☆☆☆ the most difficult. (Please note that while five-star Checkups exist, they are beyond the scope of this book. If you feel that your horse may have a problem with a five-star Checkup area, please call your certified chiropractor.)

As shown in Chart 2, there are four components to each Body Checkup, and I've rated each individually. Be aware that the overall star rating is *not* the average but is, instead, the highest star designation of the four components in the Checkup. The four components are:

CHART 1: CHALLENGE-LEVEL METHOD STAR CHECKUP CHART

☆ ONE-STAR	☆☆ TWO-STAR	☆☆☆ THREE-STAR		☆☆☆☆ FOUR-STAR	☆☆☆☆☆ FIVE-STAR
Knee Fetlock Tail	Atlas Splint Bones Withers	Accessory Carpal Bone Hip Joint Hock Intertransverse Joint Lumbar Vertebrae Neck Pastern Ribs	Sacrum Sacroiliac Joint Sesamoid Bones Shoulder Shoulder Blade Sternum Thoracic Vertebrae TMJ	C7 Coffin Joint Elbow Occiput Stifle	Cranial Bones Ear Cartilage Hyoid Bone Lumbar L6 Navicular Bone Pelvic Symphysis Ribs R1–7 Tail Vertebrae T1–T2

Five-star Checkups are listed for your information but are beyond the scope of this book.

Locating Anatomic Area: This refers to the difficulty involved in locating the anatomic area referred to in the Body Checkup directions. The more difficult it is for most people to find an area, the higher the star rating.

Positioning of Person or Horse: The more difficult or awkward the position the person (or horse) has to assume, the higher the star designation.

Subtle Range of Motion: The range of motion is the amount that a joint normally moves. When it is very small or difficult to feel, its Checkup has a higher star designation. Conversely, a large or obvious range of motion has fewer stars.

Complex Evaluation of Checkup: Sometimes you have to decide between joint movement being too small or the muscles being too tight. If the evaluation involves complicated deciphering of the body's reaction to the Checkup like this, the Checkup has a higher star designation. When it is more of a "can it move or not" (yes or no) scenario, then I've rated it lower on the scale of difficulty.

So each Body Checkup Challenge level has a lot of factors involved. Some Checkup areas are very easy to find, but have a more subtle range of motion than others. And some have an obvious range of motion, but the person is put into an awkward position.

Use this component breakdown to your advantage. For example, if you are new to horse anatomy, start out with the Checkups with only one star for Locating Anatomic Area. If you want to practice feeling the most difficult, subtle ranges of motion within a group of horses, look for Checkups with a four-star rating under Subtle Range of Motion.

CHART 2: BODY CHECKUP COMPONENT BREAKDOWN

	Accessory Carpal Bone	Atlas	C7	Coffin Joint	Elbow	Fetlock	Hip Joint	Hock	Intertrans-verse Joint	Knee	Lumbar Vertebrae	Neck	Occiput	Pastern
Locating Anatomic Part	2	1	4	1	1	1	3	1	3	1	1	2	2	1
Positioning of Person or Horse	1	2	3	1	2	1	3	2	1	1	1	2	1	1
Subtle Range of Motion	3	2	3	4	4	1	3	3	1	1	3	3	4	3
Complex Evaluation of Exam	2	2	3	3	4	1	3	3	1	1	2	3	4	1
Overall Challenge Level	☆☆☆ 3	☆☆ 2	☆☆☆☆ 4	☆☆☆☆ 4	☆☆☆☆ 4	☆ 1	☆☆☆ 3	☆☆☆ 3	☆☆☆ 3	☆ 1	☆☆☆ 3	☆☆☆ 3	☆☆☆☆ 4	☆☆☆ 3

	Ribs	Sacrum	Shoulder Blade	Sesamoid Bones	Shoulder	Sacroiliac Joint	Splint Bones	Sternum	Stifle	Tail Vertebrae	Thoracic Vertebrae	TMJ	Withers
Locating Anatomic Part	2	2	1	1	1	2	2	2	2	1	1	2	1
Positioning of Person or Horse	1	1	3	1	3	1	1	2	2	1	2	1	1
Subtle Range of Motion	2	3	2	3	2	3	3	2	2	1	3	3	2
Complex Evaluation of Exam	3	3	3	2	3	3	2	3	3	1	2	3	2
Overall Challenge Level	☆☆☆ 3	☆☆☆ 3	☆☆☆ 3	☆☆☆ 3	☆☆☆ 3	☆☆☆ 3	☆☆ 2	☆☆☆ 3	☆☆☆☆ 4	☆ 1	☆☆☆ 3	☆☆☆ 3	☆☆ 2

bug's ear together. But now Pumpkin is occasionally running out at fences. She also is giving your daughter trouble when your daughter goes to catch her—even running away from carrots! "Well, Pumpkin is 17 years old," everyone says, "Maybe it's time to retire her."

As you sit down with this book to figure out what to do, you think to yourself, "It doesn't make any sense that one week the pony was fine, and the next week she wasn't. I'm going to check things out myself."

Step One: You look through the Top 10 Complaints (p. 35), but Pumpkin's symptoms are not listed. You go on to Step Two.

Step Two: You look through the Comprehensive Complaints List (p. 161) and find Pumpkin's symptoms with corresponding Body Checkups.

As you read through the list of complaints you remember that your daughter has complained that Pumpkin is much more "bumpy" to the right when trotting. The "bumpiness" your daughter feels may have something to do with why Pumpkin prefers going to the right. You end up with the following:

Pumpkin's Symptoms

- Reluctance to jump
- Prefers one direction over the other

Pumpkin's Body Checkups: To Do

Occiput, p. 48; Atlas, p. 44; Neck, p. 56; C7, p. 60; Shoulder, p. 69; Knee, p. 81; Splint Bone, p. 87; Fetlock, p. 90; Sesamoid Bones, p. 94; Pastern, p. 98; Coffin Joint, p. 102; Thoracic Vertebrae, p. 112; Ribs, p. 117; Lumbar Vertebrae, p. 122; Sacrum, p. 130; Sacroiliac Joint, p. 134; Stifle, p. 141; Hock, p. 145

Because this Body Checkup list is so long anyway, you decide to go ahead and check all the areas of the pony. You think to yourself, "This is just the kick in the pants I need to learn this stuff. I'm going to learn it all perfectly!"

You do a great job with your Body Checkups, but are now scratching your head with the results. You were expecting to find a lot wrong with Pumpkin, since she is 17 years old, after all. But the only Checkups where you've found probable subluxations are:

- Atlas
- Lumbar vertebrae
- Right sacroiliac joint
- Right hock

Since you found four probable subluxations, you call the chiropractor out. The chiropractor tells you that you are amazing! Which, of course, you are. A few days after the adjustment, your daughter tells you that Pumpkin is definitely less "bumpy." However, she is still running out at fences, and still doesn't want to be caught—although she will now come up and eat the carrots, so at least there's that.

You redo your exams, being very picky now. All you can find this time is a possible right hock subluxation. "Well," you reason, "I know this right hock is not working right, but I guess I don't know how bad it really is, since all I'm comparing it to is Pumpkin's left hock." So you ask some of the other owners at the barn if you can check out their ponies so you can get a really good feel for hock movement.

As you recheck Pumpkin's hocks after checking several other ponies, you realize that the left one doesn't move correctly, and the right one doesn't move at all. "Perfect!" you think to yourself, "Now I know what to do."

You call your vet and get a consultation on Pumpkin's hocks. Your vet believes injections are the way to go, followed by an intramuscular joint supplement. Once Pumpkin's joints get the lubrication they need, Pumpkin is happy to be caught and jump once again.

Were the hocks the primary problem? Could you have skipped the chiropractor all together? In this situation, it didn't matter who was called first. Both the veterinarian (to inject the hocks to fix the reluctance to jump) and the chiropractor (to correct Pumpkin's preferring to go in one direction—exhibited as "bumpiness) were needed.

Example Three

A Simple Answer

Now that your barn friends know that you're an expert in finding out where a horse hurts, they start asking you questions. One woman gets out the journal she keeps, with notes on her horse's lameness problem, and starts reading it to you. Before your eyes glazed completely over, you ask her: "Is the lameness more obvious at the walk or the trot?"

"Oh," she replies. "It's always worse at the walk, which, I think, is why the trainer thinks I'm crazy. That and the fact that I have this journal."

"If it is more obvious at the walk," you respond, "your best bet is to start with the certified chiropractor. Nothing is 100 percent, but it's most often a chiropractic issue when the problem is worse at the walk."

"Wow!" the woman exclaims. "You have just saved me weeks of figuring this out and lots of money in vet bills! Let me take you out to dinner!"

Body Checkups: Final Instructions (and Caveats)

The 27 Body Checkups are divided into four sections to cover the horse's entire body by starting at the head and finishing at the tail: the Head and Neck (five Checkups, p. 43); the Front End (eleven Checkups, p. 65); the Back (five Checkups, p. 107); and the Hind End (six Checkups, p. 129).

Each Checkup is organized in a similar manner and contains the following information:

COMMON SYMPTOMS

These are some of the symptoms you may see when a joint in question is subluxated. I have organized each Checkup's list of common symptoms under the headings: Very Common; Frequent; and Occasional. Remember these only pertain to the "average" horse, and your horse may show one, some, or all of these symptoms, or he may show an Occasional symptom all the time.

(NOTE: When your horse has a subluxated joint that is a secondary subluxation brought on by a primary cause—rather than a primary chiropractic issue—your horse may show *none* of these symptoms. See more about primary causes on p. 19.)

FUNCTION

This section gives a brief summary of the most common functions for the body part you are checking. All body parts have multiple functions. The functions mentioned here are the ones most applicable to the Checkup.

NORMAL RANGE OF MOTION

"Range of motion" is the term used for how a body part normally moves. Since you will be checking range of motion of a joint or vertebra, you need to know its normal parameters. Please note, however, that all bones and vertebra move in three dimensions. The Body Checkups covered in this book are described in a two-dimensional manner for ease of communication.

HOW TO—TESTING AND DIAGNOSING

There are always many ways to check the same body part. The methods I describe are the ones that I use every day and find easiest for most people to learn.

The accompanying photos show what a close-up of the anatomical part you are examining will look like, as well as an idea of how you should stand, and how your horse should be positioned. You may have to "tweak" your own stance depending on your size, and your horse's. Don't be concerned if your position doesn't look exactly like the person's in the sample photos. You are free to move however you need to so that you and your horse are comfortable.

SUMMARY

Each summary analyzes the Checkup's results. It includes a list of "additional possibilities" to consider when you fail to find evidence of subluxation. This list, not in any special order, contains the most commonly seen "other causes," but it is not all-inclusive.

Lastly, in the summary I make some suggestions about what to do when you find a problem in the area you are checking. Just remember, these are only "suggestions." Do what your gut instinct tells you to do.

Section 1

THE HEAD AND NECK BODY CHECKUPS

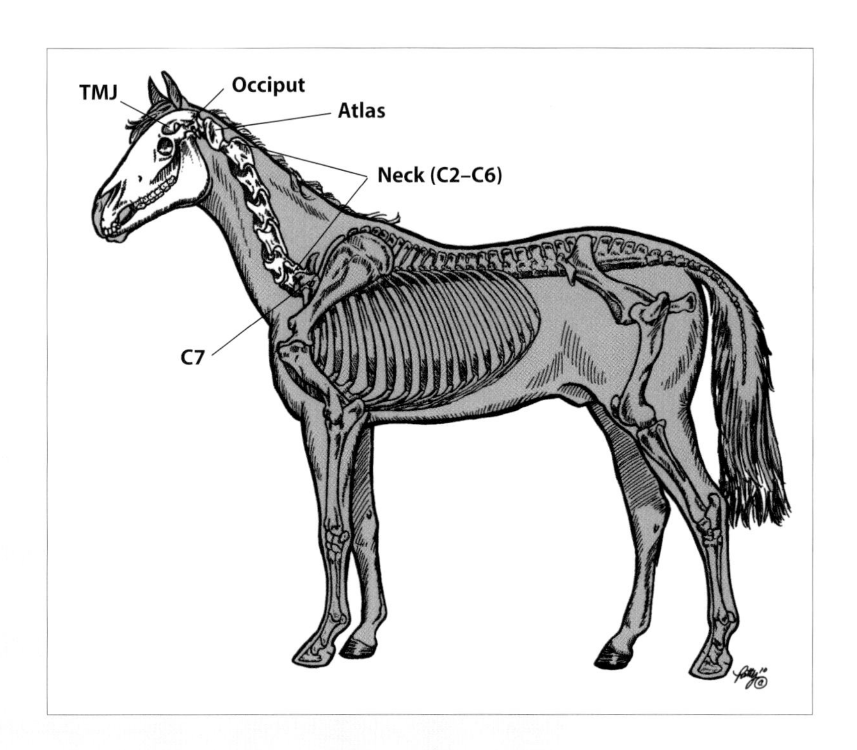

The Head and Neck Body Checkup areas.

Head and Neck Problems: General Symptoms

- Difficulty picking up, maintaining, or changing leads
- Difficulty with poll flexion
- Uncomfortable with haltering and/or bridling
- Having an obviously favorite lead
- Head-shy
- Ear-shy
- Tips nose to the outside when doing circle work
- Bracing on or evading the bit, especially one side only
- Inability to focus or concentrate
- Spooky
- Standoffish, non-affectionate
- Facial expression that often indicates: "I have a headache. Don't bother me."
- Inability to do "long-and-low" work comfortably
- Difficulty with collection or impulsion
- Stiff neck or body
- Inability to bend neck right or left
- Unwilling to open mouth for bit
- Difficulty chewing on one or both sides

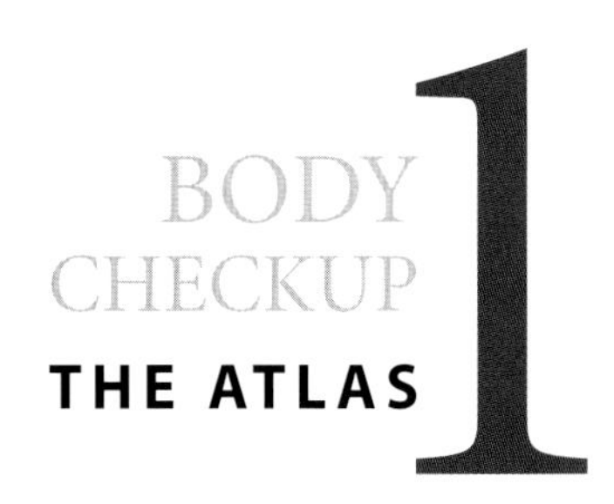

BODY CHECKUP 1 THE ATLAS

Jag was a 10-year-old sorrel Quarter Horse. My longtime clients, Jenny and Gene, called to have me take a look at him. They had been in the horse-training business for over 30 years. They said to me, "If you can't fix him, we'll have to put him down. He's too dangerous."

"Why? What on earth happened?" I asked in astonishment.

Jenny replied, "That horse came after Gene like he was going to take him out. I mean, full gallop, teeth bared, ears flat back. Gene tried to call his bluff, only he wasn't bluffing. Usually a horse will turn aside if you stand your ground, but Jag kept coming and hit Gene in the chest! If Gene hadn't finally jumped out of the way, Jag would have run him over."

I could hardly believe my ears—Gene was a true horse expert. He could normally read horses perfectly from 100 feet away. "Do you know what set him off?" I asked.

"Anytime you try to do anything around his head he starts getting that evil look in his eye," replied Jenny.

Well, with a few Body Checkups I discovered that Jag's atlas was subluxated—the farthest I had ever seen. One side was easily 3 inches off from the other. I can't imagine the kind of pain that horse was suffering. I was able to adjust it, although we had to use a twitch with two men holding him for safety.

The very next day Jenny called in tears. "What's going on?" I asked. Jenny said that Jag had put his head out over the stall door, which he never does, and when she came over to him, he did something new: He turned his head toward her. "It was like he wanted me to touch his face," Jenny said. "So I did, and he was perfectly happy letting me pet him all over his head. He never got that evil look in his eye at all! It's a miracle!"

ATLAS CHALLENGE LEVEL ☆☆
Locating Anatomic Area: ☆
Positioning of Person or Horse: ☆☆
Subtle Range of Motion: ☆☆
Complex Evaluation of Checkup: ☆☆

Common Symptoms

BEHAVIORAL OR PERFORMANCE SYMPTOMS

Very Common

- Difficulty picking up or maintaining leads
- Difficulty with poll flexion
- Having an obviously favorite lead

Frequent

- Head-shy
- Uncomfortable with haltering and/or bridling
- Ear-shy
- Tips nose to the outside when doing circle work
- Unable to do "long-and-low" work comfortably
- Difficulty with collection or impulsion

Occasional

- Unable to focus or concentrate
- Spooky
- Standoffish or not affectionate
- Facial expression that often indicates: "I have a headache. Don't bother me."
- Bracing on or evading the bit, especially one side only

PHYSICAL SYMPTOMS: CURRENT OR PRIOR

- Dental problems—especially asymmetrical tooth wear
- Poll, tight muscles around it
- TMJ issues
- Ewe neck

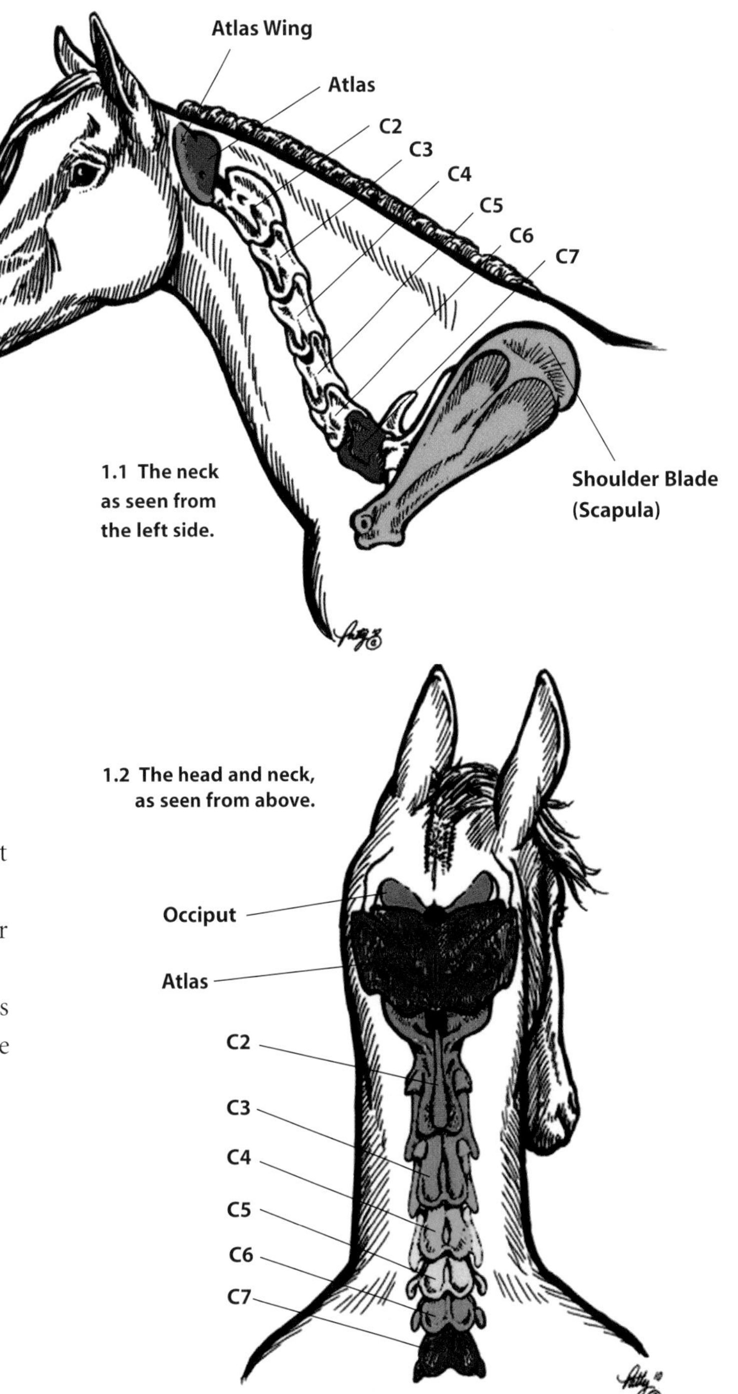

1.1 The neck as seen from the left side.

1.2 The head and neck, as seen from above.

Checkup Directions

FUNCTION: The atlas, also called the poll or the first cervical vertebra (C1), is one of the two anchor points for the dura mater of the spinal cord; the other anchor point is the sacrum. The atlas is responsible for 90 percent of the head's rotational movement. It is also protection for the brainstem as it travels from the skull to the remainder of the spinal column.

NORMAL RANGE OF MOTION: The atlas can move quite a bit in order to rotate the horse's nose right or left. It easily moves 1 to 2 inches as it is pulled down toward the ground on each side, and also moves from front to back (toward the tail) approximately one-quarter inch.

HOW TO

Stand facing the rear of the horse. Stand either directly under the horse's head, or to his side, whichever is more comfortable for you. The atlas sits under the headstall of the halter. Place your hands on each side of the horse's atlas, sliding down from midline onto the wings of the atlas (fig. 1.3).

TEST 1

The wings of the atlas may be up to 6 inches long, so don't worry about exactly where your fingers are; just place them in approximately the same spot on both sides of the horse (fig. 1.4). Hopefully, the horse is comfortable with where you and your hands are located. Some horses can become concerned with your position and tense up. Just give him time to relax. If he doesn't, consider his actions part of your diagnosis.

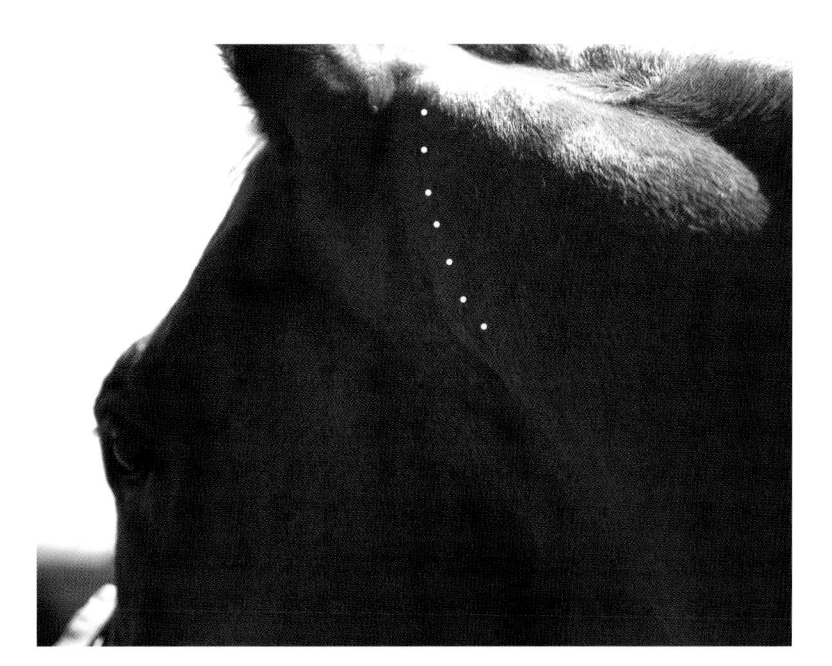

1.3 The side view of the atlas area. The edge of the atlas wings are marked by the white dots.

TEST 2

With your fingers still on the wings of the atlas, gently pull one side of the atlas down toward the ground. Release the atlas as you come to its natural stopping point. Pull down and release on that side a few times to get a feel for the atlas' range of motion. The horse's head should rotate along with the atlas. Repeat this on the other side. The atlas should move the same distance down toward the ground on both sides, and without tension or resistance.

1.4 In this photo, the atlas wings are level, as indicated by my index fingers.

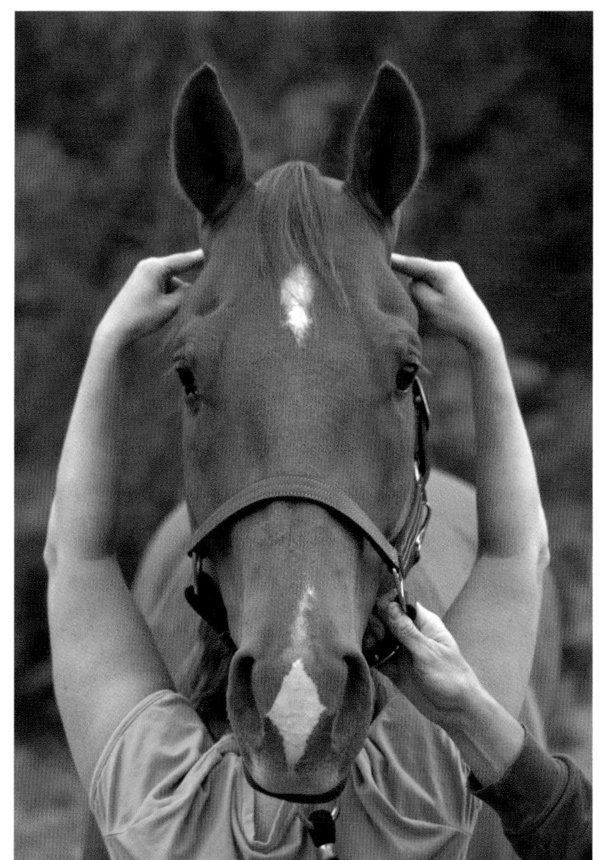

Diagnosis

If the horse is evasive (especially with your hand placement), the area has probably become sensitive to touch and it's highly likely that the atlas is subluxated. Also, when you place your hands on both sides of the atlas wings and your fingers sit higher on one side than the other, you can be pretty certain the atlas is subluxated (fig. 1.5). When both sides of the atlas do not move through their range of motion with the same ease and for the same distance, the atlas is subluxated. Of course, the atlas could be "stuck" evenly on both sides. You need experience working with different horses to determine if this is the case.

1.5 Here the horse's atlas is higher on his left side, as you can see by my right index finger, which is higher than the left finger.

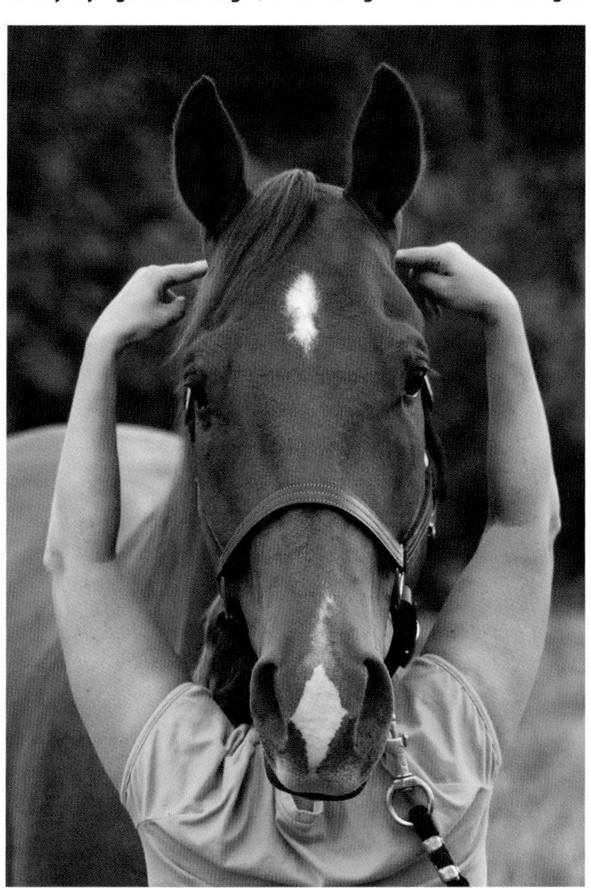

An interesting fact about the atlas is that it works together—functionally—with the occiput and TMJ (temporomandibular joint). I call it the "TMJ-atlas-occiput triangle." You can feel part of this "triangle action" on yourself with a simple experiment: Tip your head to one side, relax and wait a minute. You'll feel your jaw (TMJ) move over to the same side as your head. This test shows you the body's interconnections in a small way.

When any one of the three points of the triangle is subluxated, it tends to pull the other two parts out of alignment with it. Be sure to check the TMJ (p. 52) and occiput (p. 48) when you feel the atlas is subluxated.

Summary: ATLAS

- When indication of probable subluxation, call chiropractor.
- No subluxation, check for other causes of atlas symptoms:
    - Chiropractic subluxations at: occiput, TMJ, or C2 (pp. 48, 52, 56)
    - Dental problems, sharp tooth edges, or tooth abscesses
    - Mouth ulcerations
    - Bit discomfort
    - Guttural pouch infection
    - Sinus infection
    - Gluten sensitivity (when horse shows inability to concentrate)

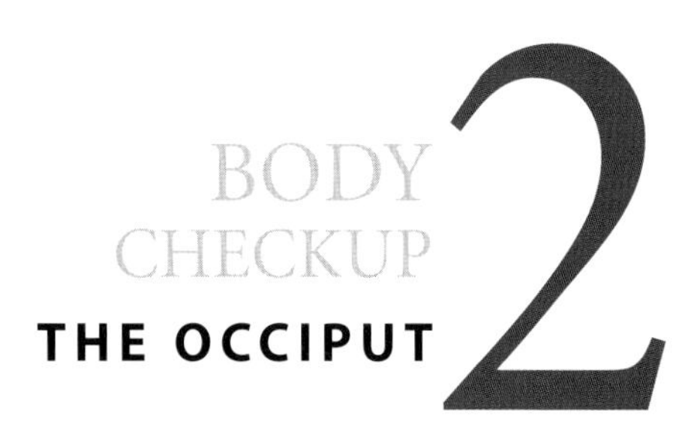

One warm sunny day I was at a dressage barn to do a chiropractic exam on a five-year-old Oldenberg gelding. He was bay, charming, and really lovely—if you don't mind my using that term when referring to a gelding.

Anyway, Clare, his new owner, was having trouble getting his poll to flex and had him adjusted several times by different chiropractors over the past few months. Each time helped, but only briefly. Before I got started with the exam, I asked his name.

"Oh, his name is Spitty," Clare answered.

"What?" I said. "This beautiful boy is named Spitty?"

Clare replied, "Well, actually, his name is Reginald III, but we all call him Spitty. It's because of how he drools and spits all over when he's ridden." I asked her to clarify, because it was my understanding that most dressage riders want to see some saliva or a "frothy mouth" when a horse is being ridden.

"They do!" Clare said. "But Spitty has soooo much spit! And way more on one side of his mouth than the other. He also used to constantly chew on the bit…a lot. So I put a dropped noseband on him—and, wouldn't you know, now he sticks his tongue out the side of his mouth! The same side as the drool!"

As I went over Spitty's body, I found his atlas to be subluxated along with his TMJ. But more importantly, I found that his occiput was also subluxated. And I was glad to find this. You see, sometimes an atlas continuously re-subluxates when the occiput and/or TMJ are also subluxated but not corrected. In Spitty's case, once his entire head was adjusted, rather than just his atlas, he was able to flex his poll, his atlas stopped subluxating on a regular basis, and he even stopped spitting! Clare was able to remove the dropped noseband and ride a much happier horse. (But she still calls him Spitty.)

A lot of horses get their atlas adjusted—this is important because the spinal cord runs through it. On occasion, however, I have run into clients who tell me their horse needs to have his atlas adjusted every month. *This should not be necessary.* The atlas and the sacrum are "anchor points" for the spinal cord; the dura mater of the spinal cord *only* attaches at the atlas and sacrum (see pp. 44 and 130). If one or both of these areas become subluxated, it creates subluxations up and down the spine.

If your horse requires repeated atlas adjusting, be sure to check the occiput. The occiput, TMJ

OCCIPUT CHALLENGE LEVEL ★★★★
Locating Anatomic Area: ★★
Positioning of Person or Horse: ★
Subtle Range of Motion: ★★★★
Complex Evaluation of Checkup: ★★★★

(p. 52) and atlas work in a *triangular* fashion. When one corner of the triangle is subluxated, it puts strain on the other two corners, which then may also become subluxated. Therefore, if the entire "triangle" is not corrected, but only one corner, the problem will return.

Check dental floating history with recurrent "triangle" subluxations, as teeth imbalances can also cause subluxations of the atlas, occiput, and/or TMJ.

Common Symptoms

BEHAVIORAL AND PERFORMANCE SYMPTOMS

*Very Common**

- Difficulty picking up or maintaining leads
- Difficulty with poll flexion

Frequent

- Ear-shy
- Difficulty changing leads

Occasional

- Difficulty with poll flexion
- Head or nose tilted to one side when riding or longeing
- Bracing on a rein or evading the bit, especially one side only
- Difficulty bending neck, especially upper neck
- Head-shy
- Uncomfortable with haltering or bridling
- Spooky
- Standoffish or not affectionate

*(*It is rare for the occiput to be subluxated alone. These very common symptoms typically occur when the atlas is also subluxated.)*

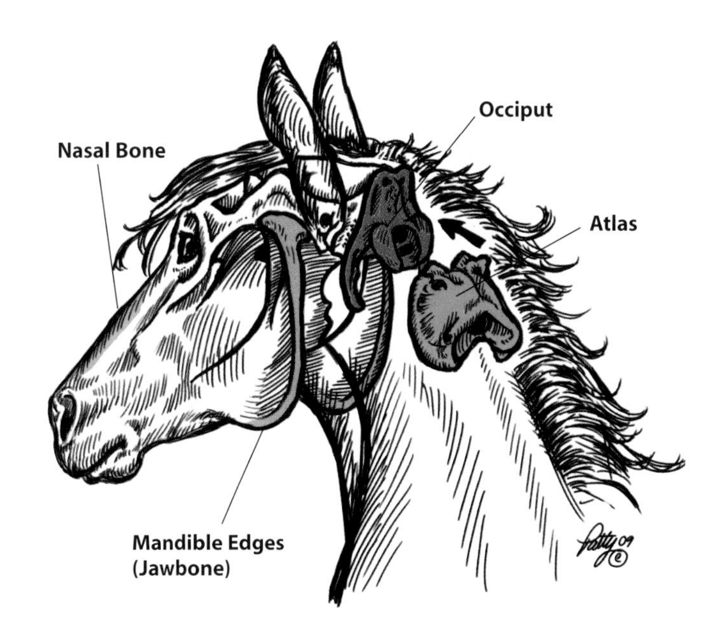

2.1 The head of the horse as seen at an angle from the side. The occiput and atlas together compose the atlanto-occipital joint. This drawing shows the atlas and occiput separated in order to give a clear view of the occiput though normally the atlas sits right up next to the occiput, as indicated by the black arrow. The skull, for naming purposes, is divided into several sections. The occiput is the name of the rear section of the skull.

PHYSICAL SYMPTOMS: CURRENT OR PRIOR

- Atlas chronically subluxates
- Dental problems, especially asymmetrical tooth wear
- TMJ issues
- Poll surrounded by tight muscles
- Ewe neck

Checkup Directions

FUNCTION: The *occiput* is the name for the back part of the horse's skull—it is positioned right in front of the atlas. Its connection with the atlas, which

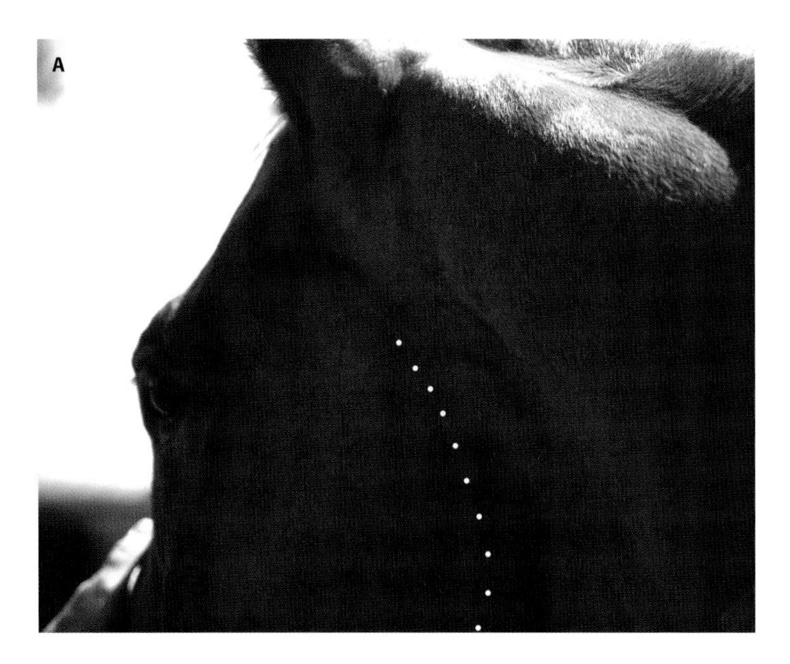

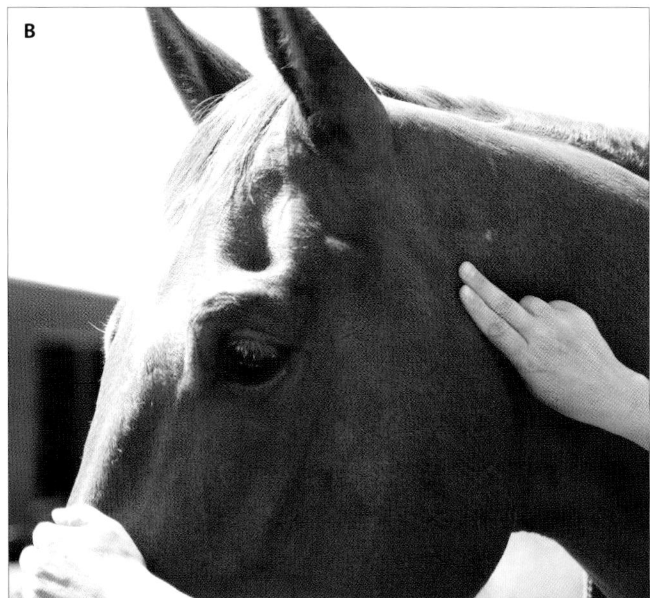

2.2 A & B When checking the occiput, place the fingers of one hand between the mandible (marked with white dots in A) and the atlas wing (B).

is called the *atlanto-occipital joint,* enables the horse to move his head in all directions. The brain stem also emerges from the occiput, which is one reason why the atlanto-occipital connection is so important at the top of the spinal column.

NORMAL RANGE OF MOTION: The normal range of motion of the occiput is a left-to-right and up-and-down movement of the head *without any* movement of the neck. This movement is very small—approximately 15 degrees in each direction. If the head is moved past 15 degrees, the neck automatically becomes involved in the the occiput's movement.

HOW TO

Place one or two fingers between the mandible (jawbone) and the wing of the atlas (figs. 2.2 A & B).

Place the other hand lightly across the front of the horse's nose, holding gently onto the nasal bone. Use the nose to flex the head right and left, while using very light finger pressure to keep the neck from moving (fig. 2.3).

This flexing should be gentle and small—less than an inch of movement from the hand on the nose. Too much force causes the horse's muscles to tense, so to avoid this, immediately after you flex in one direction, release the nose. As you flex and release, then flex and release again, the movement becomes a bit like a gentle "bounce" of the head from center to side.

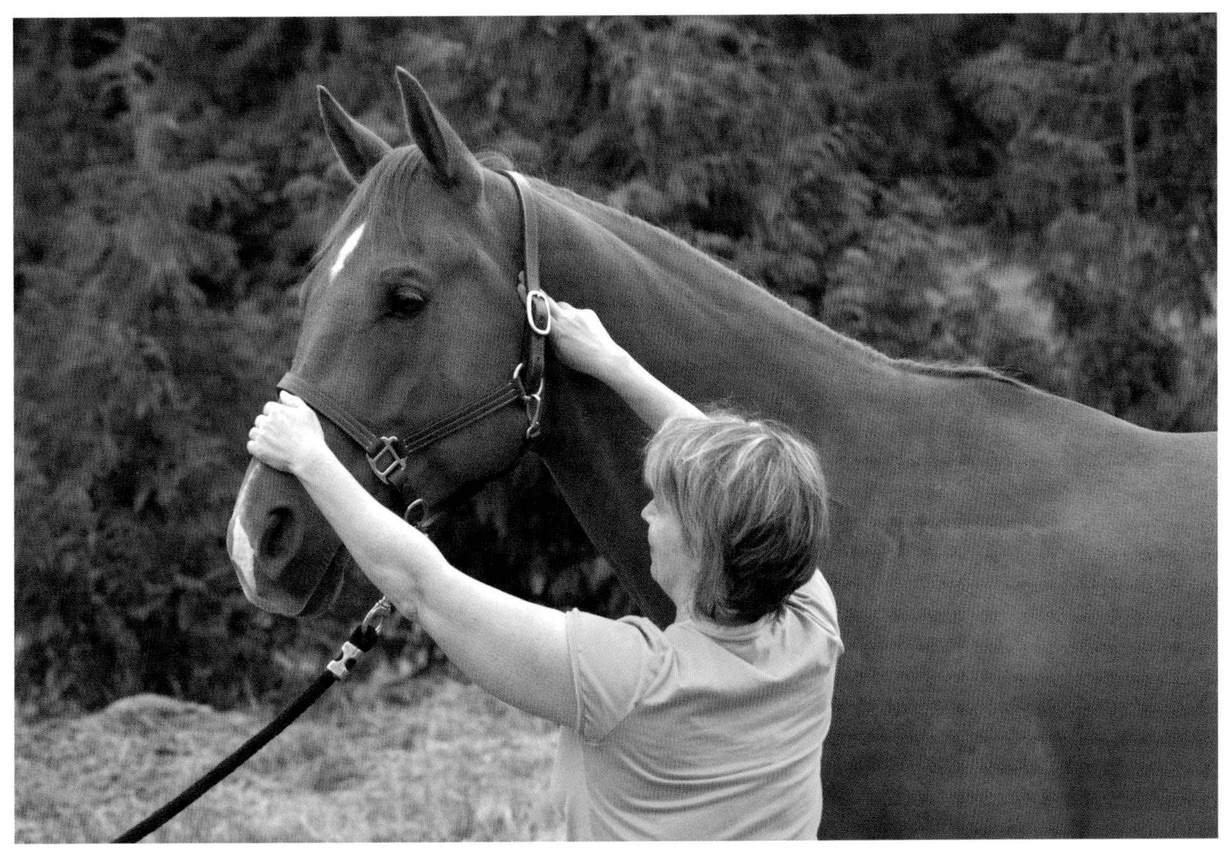

2.3 The occiput Checkup is a subtle movement.

Diagnosis

Check the ability of the head to move both right and left. It should flex easily about 15 degrees in both directions. When the occiput flexes easily (or "bounces") to one side but not to the other, the occiput is subluxated.

Summary: OCCIPUT

- When subluxation indicated, call chiropractor.
- No subluxation: Check for these other possible causes of occiput symptoms:
    - Chiropractic subluxations at: atlas, TMJ (pp. 44 and 52)
    - Dental problems
    - Bit discomfort

BODY CHECKUP 3
THE TMJ
(Temporomandibular Joint)

Ulysses was a 33-year-old Arabian stallion whose elderly owner simply wanted to do everything possible to keep her "boy" healthy and happy. We did chiropractic and acupuncture treatments on his "spa day" every couple of months, which he thoroughly enjoyed. He needed very few chiropractic adjustments each time, except for one chronic TMJ. I'd regularly ask her these same questions:

Have his teeth been floated recently?

Yes, the "teeth guy" comes every six months.

Does he eat okay? Drop his feed?

No, he eats just fine.

She didn't ride him, so my usual "leaning-on-a-rein" and "stiff-neck" questions weren't applicable.

Despite her answers, the horse's TMJ pain response was slowly but surely getting worse. I finally got a clue when I tried to check his teeth myself. I simply placed my fingers at his lips, and he raised his head to avoid me, then suddenly started shaking his head and backing up rapidly. "How long has he been doing *that*?" I asked.

"Oh, he never likes his mouth looked at," his owner said. "They always tranquilize him first to check his teeth." My inner alarm went off at this information, particularly since I knew Ulysses to be extremely well behaved in every other instance.

I strongly encouraged Ulysses' owner to have a professional veterinary dentist look at her horse's teeth. It actually took me several more visits to convince her, mostly because she had used her "teeth guy" for many years and was very loyal. However, when Ulysses was finally examined by another tooth professional, he was found to have dental hooks on his *lower* teeth in the very back of his mouth that were so long (over 2 inches!) that they poked him in the *upper* jaw. No wonder he never let anyone try to open his mouth—opening his mouth *hurt!*

Once Ulysses had his teeth floated by a professional equine dentist, his TMJ pain left immediately. He still continues to enjoy his "spa treatments" on a regular basis.

TMJ CHALLENGE LEVEL ☆☆☆
Locating Anatomic Area: ☆☆
Positioning of Person or Horse: ☆
Subtle Range of Motion: ☆☆☆
Complex Evaluation of Checkup: ☆☆☆

Common Symptoms

BEHAVIORAL AND PERFORMANCE SYMPTOMS

Very Common

- Bracing on a rein or evading the bit, especially one side only
- Unable to open mouth wide

Frequent

- Unwilling to open mouth for bit
- Difficulty chewing on one or both sides of the mouth

Occasional

- Head-shy
- Ear-shy
- Difficulty flexing poll
- Difficulty bending right or left at poll

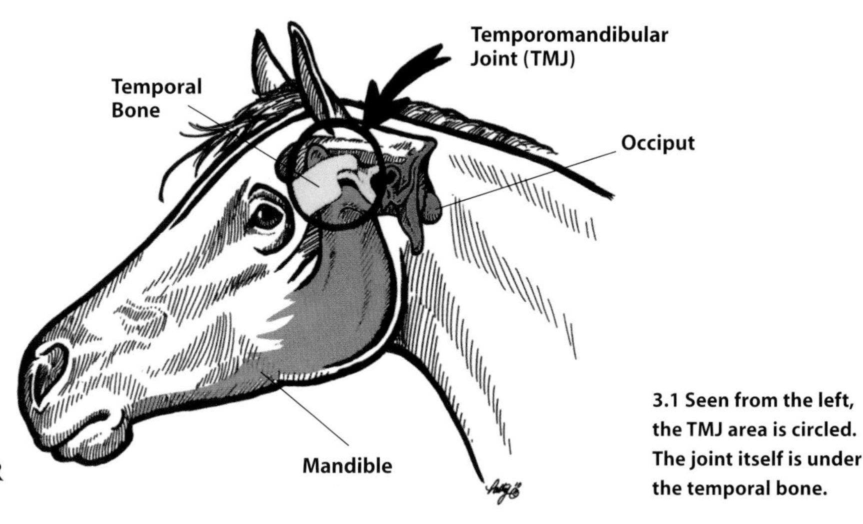

3.1 Seen from the left, the TMJ area is circled. The joint itself is under the temporal bone.

PHYSICAL SYMPTOMS: CURRENT OR PRIOR

- Atlas subluxations
- Occiput subluxations
- Sacroiliac subluxations
- Dental problems, history of
- Poll, tight muscles surrounding it

Checkup Directions

FUNCTION: There are two temporomandibular (TMJ) joints, one on the left and one on the right side of the jaw. The TMJ joints allow for the opening and closing of the mouth as well as the chewing of food. The primary function of the TMJ is the opening and closing of the jaw. In addition, it is the joint with the highest number of proprioceptive nerves in the entire body. This means that the TMJ also functions as a "balancing station," telling the horse where his body is in space.

NORMAL RANGE OF MOTION: To get an idea of the TMJ's normal range of motion, open and close your own jaw and also move your lower jaw side to side. TMJ movement in the horse is very similar. You can check the side-to-side movement of the horse's TMJ, as well as for any pain in the TMJ area. Measured at the incisor area, the lower jaw should be able to slide right and left approximately one-half inch—at a minimum—with no resistance.

HOW TO

TEST 1

Check the range of motion of the TMJ by moving the lower jaw (mandible) *gently* from side to side. It should slide easily in a relaxed manner the same distance to the right as to the left. The best hand position to use is with one hand on the nose (not the halter) to keep the head still, while your other hand cups the lower jaw (fig. 3.2). Your lower hand slides the jaw slowly and gently,

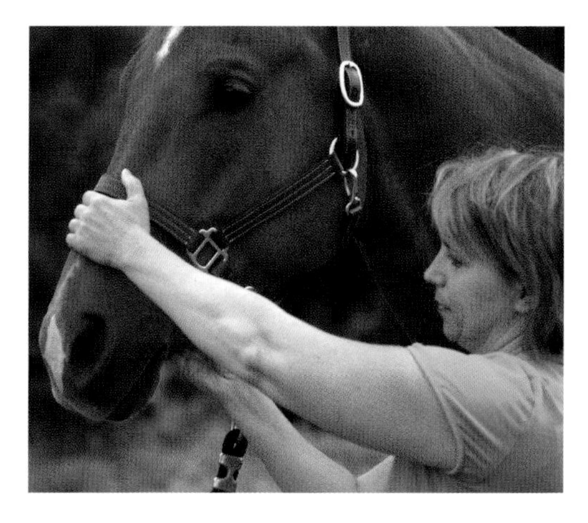

3.2 The TMJ Checkup position.

A

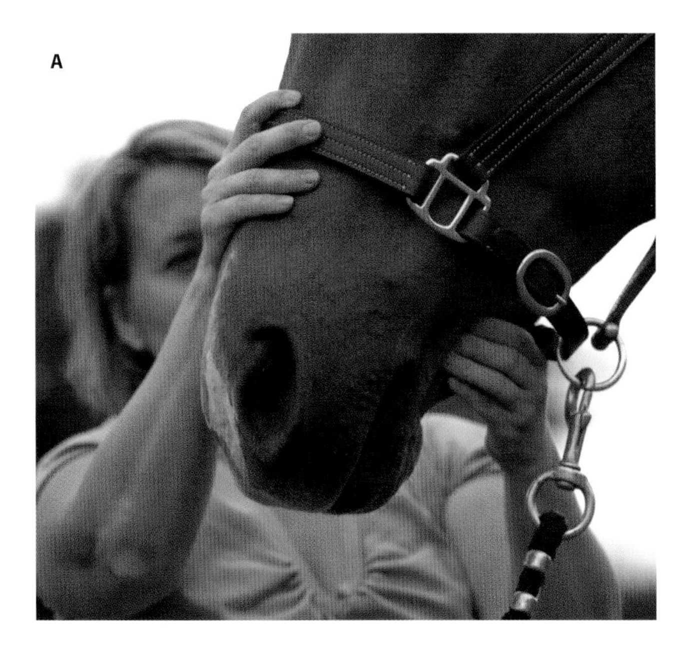

B

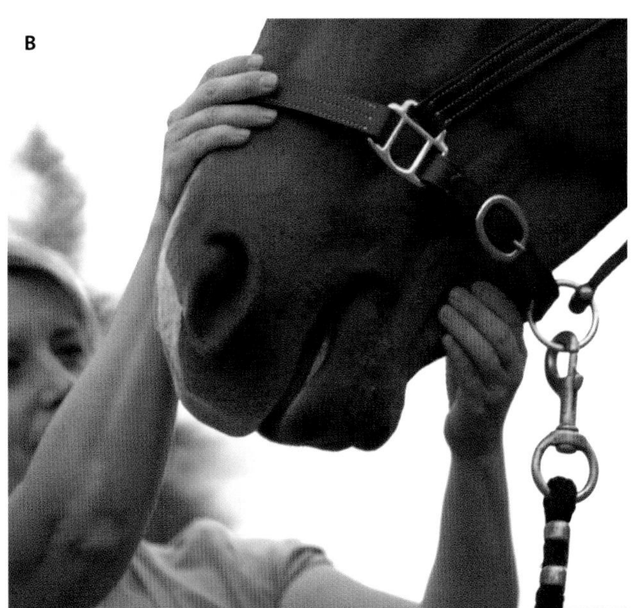

3.3 A & B I demonstrate sliding the horse's lower jaw from side to side. In photo B, note how the lower jaw has moved over to the horse's left approximately one-half inch.

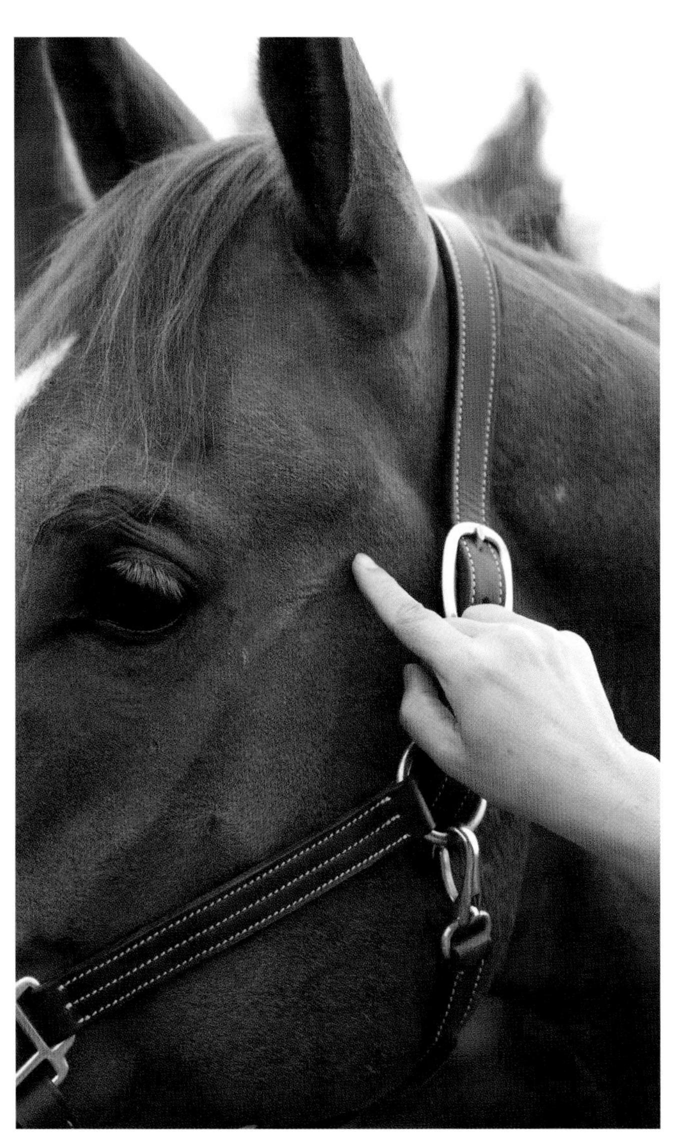

3.4 When checking the muscles and ligaments of the TMJ area, you must press *gently*.

first to one side and then the other (figs. 3.3 A & B). Make sure the horse's entire head does not tip side to side, instead of the lower jaw moving independently of the head.

TEST 2

Another Checkup is to press on the associated muscles and ligaments of the TMJ to see if they are sensitive (fig. 3.4). It is extremely important to *press gently,* especially at first. As mentioned, the TMJ contains many nerves, so when it is subluxated, it can be so sore the horse may react violently with a sudden swing of the head toward you. When the TMJ is normal, you should be able to push the TMJ area with the same amount of pressure that you can push on your own TMJ and not feel any pain.

Diagnosis

If the TMJ movement is not smooth and easy; not symmetrical (traveling the same distance both right and left); or the TMJ area is tender to the touch, it is likely that one or both TMJ joints are subluxated. NOTE: It is also possible that there are teeth issues, such as floating needs, which should be addressed before the TMJ is adjusted.

Check the Whole Triangle

The TMJ functions within the *TMJ-atlas-occiput triangle* (p. 49). When one of these three is subluxated, it usually affects the other two. Always check all three, when you are suspicious of any one of these areas.

Summary: TMJ

- When one—or all—indications of subluxation are present and, the horse's teeth have already been checked by an equine dentist, call chiropractor.
- When no subluxation indicated, yet symptoms of a TMJ problem remain, check for:
  - Chiropractic subluxations at: atlas, occiput, neck (C2–C6)—pp. 44, 48, 56
  - Dental problems requiring floating
  - Tooth abscess
  - Bit discomfort
  - Neck muscle issues
  - Heavy-handed riding

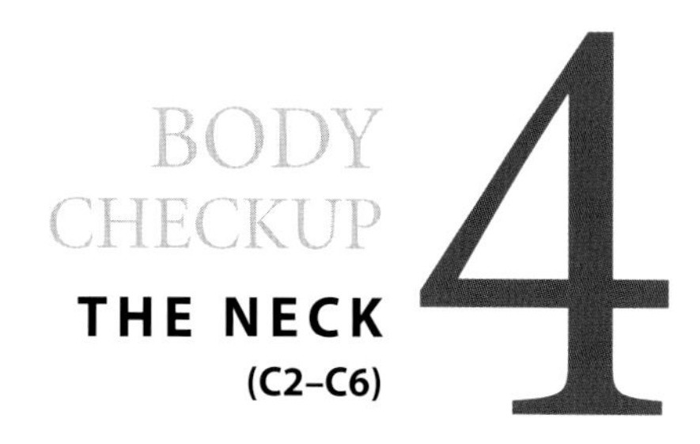

A five-year-old, 17.2-hand Thoroughbred gelding named Ben continually got a subluxation in the right side of his neck, making it very difficult for him to bend to the right. We had to adjust his neck once a month, which is really too often, especially for such a young horse. And every month, there was nothing else chiropractically wrong with him.

His teeth were good and he had no history of injury. It was a bit perplexing. It actually bothered me a lot more than it did the owner. She was just happy he could be "fixed" and that I was willing to come out every month. Perhaps that was why it took some time before I finally learned from the caretaker that Ben was always sticking his head and neck through the fence to eat. Mind you, he's out in a 10-acre pasture with plenty of grass. (This proves that the grass really is greener on the other side of the fence!)

Just because a horse sticks his head through a fence does not necessarily mean his neck will subluxate all the time. However, when he's in this position and his best buddy comes up and bites him on the behind, he's asking for trouble as he jerks his neck back through the rails to defend himself. Ah, horses.

NECK CHALLENGE LEVEL ☆☆☆
Locating Anatomic Area: ☆☆
Positioning of Person or Horse: ☆☆
Subtle Range of Motion: ☆☆☆
Complex Evaluation of Checkup: ☆☆☆

Common Symptoms

BEHAVIORAL OR PERFORMANCE SYMPTOMS

Very Common

- Stiff neck or body
- Unable to bend neck right or left
- Difficulty with collection or impulsion
- Unable to do "long-and-low" work
- Bracing on a rein

Frequent

- Goes wide on turns
- Drops shoulder on turns
- Reluctant to bend body

Occasional

- Stiff in the front end
- Uncomfortable with haltering or bridling

PHYSICAL SYMPTOM: CURRENT OR PRIOR

- Ewe neck

Checkup Directions

FUNCTION: Neck (cervical) vertebrae enable movement of the neck, both right to left, and up and down.

NORMAL RANGE OF MOTION: The neck vertebrae have some of the widest range of motion in the entire body. They can move up and down, side to side, as well as twist. You will check the vertebrae at the position where the bones most easily rotate.

HOW TO

As you go down the cervical spine, after the atlas there are five cervical vertebrae (numbered C2–C6) that can be felt. These are located on the side of the neck in the lower segment of the widest part of the neck (figs. 4.3 A & B). All the neck muscles are above these vertebrae. For a few minutes, practice feeling the spaces between the vertebrae: As you run your hand along them, you'll feel a hard area (a vertebra) followed by a slight drop into a small soft spot (a joint). This is immediately followed by another vertebra.

Check each vertebra at the point where it has the greatest movement. In order to do this, the horse's neck must be curved toward you, which eliminates some of its ability to move. This way you can isolate the vertebra you want to check. The horse's head should be shifted over 1 to 2 feet while the neck curves, as if you are doing a partial carrot stretch (fig. 4.4).

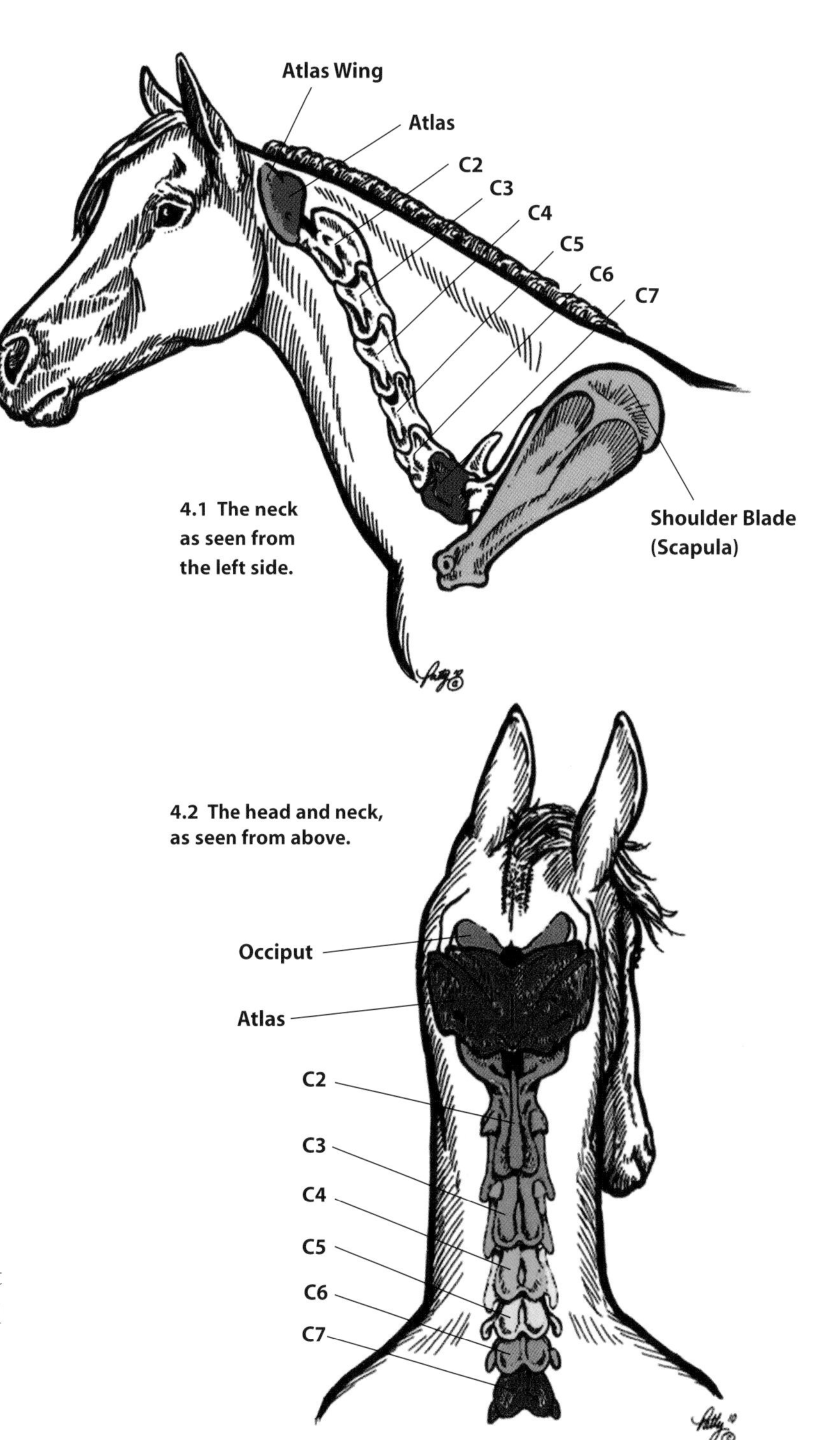

4.1 The neck as seen from the left side.

4.2 The head and neck, as seen from above.

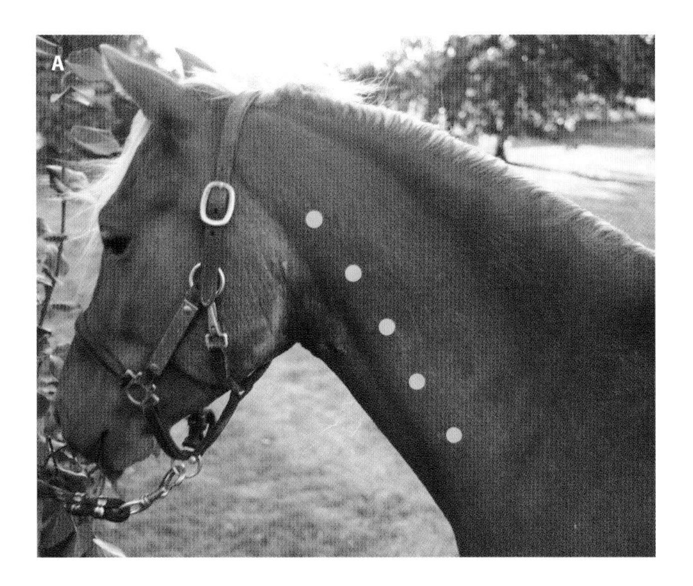

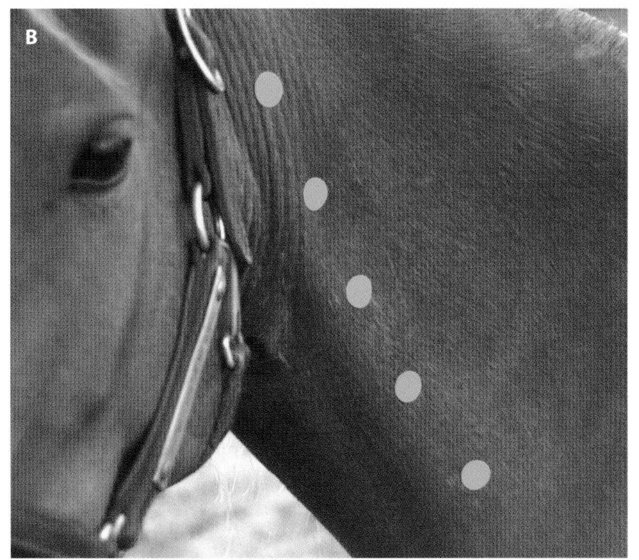

4.3 A & B The green dots in both these photos mark the spaces in between each neck vertebra, seen from different angles. Note that the neck vertebrae are found in the lower segment of the neck.

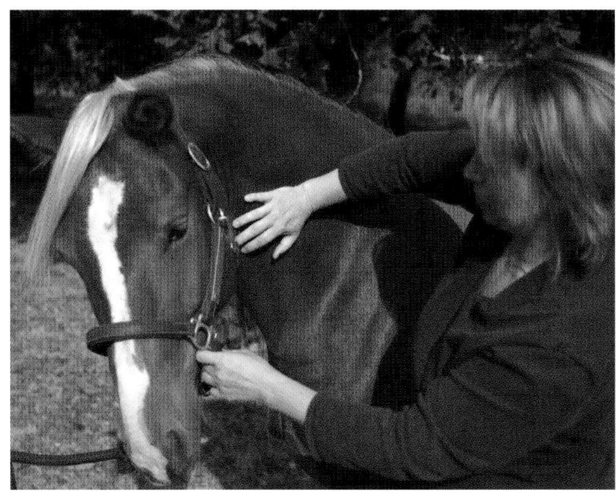

4.4 Here, the horse's head is gently curved around to the left as I perform the neck Checkup.

Place your fingers lightly under the halter to ask the horse to curve his neck to the side. It is important not to use force to pull the neck because that causes neck muscles to tighten, which will interfere with the neck Checkup.

Run your hand along the horse's neck, and when you get a feel for where each vertebra is located, check it as follows:

Place the pisiform section of your hand on the center of an individual neck vertebra (fig. 4.5 A). Gently push down at approximately a 45-degree angle from the top of the neck (fig. 4.5 B). Your elbow will point upward to create this angle. Depending on your height—and the horse's—you may need to use a step stool in order to be at the correct angle. As you push down, the vertebra should move down at least one inch. Use the amount of pressure that you would use to massage the top of your own forearm.

Diagnosis

You are looking for a "bounce" to the bone as it moves downward: It should move down with your hand pressure and come back up (this is the "bounce") when you release the pressure. If, instead, it feels as if your hand is pressing against an immoveable rock, you are feeling a subluxation. This "rock" feeling is literally as if you're pressing on solid bone, with no "give" at all. Be sure to check both sides of the neck. One side may feel perfectly "bouncy," while the other side feels like rocks.

Another sign of a subluxation is when you find the horse is repeatedly sensitive to the area you are checking.

Summary: NECK

- When either, or both, subluxation indications found, call chiropractor.
- No chiropractic issues found, but symptoms of a neck problem remain, check for:
  - Chiropractic subluxations at: withers, ribs, lumbar area (pp. 108, 117, 122)
  - TMJ or dental issues
  - Bit discomfort
  - Neck abscess, either chronic or acute (caused by vaccine or bug bite, for example)

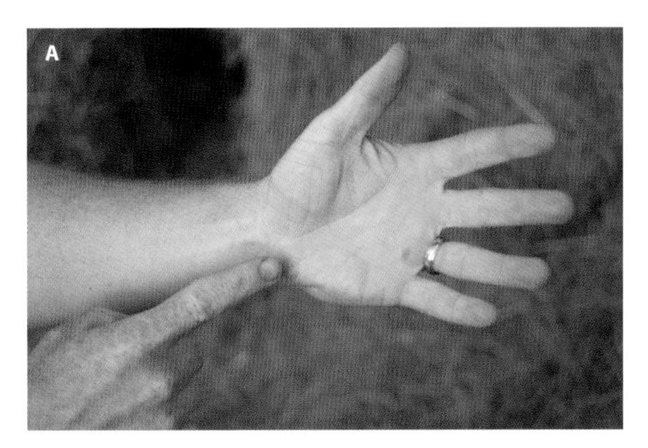

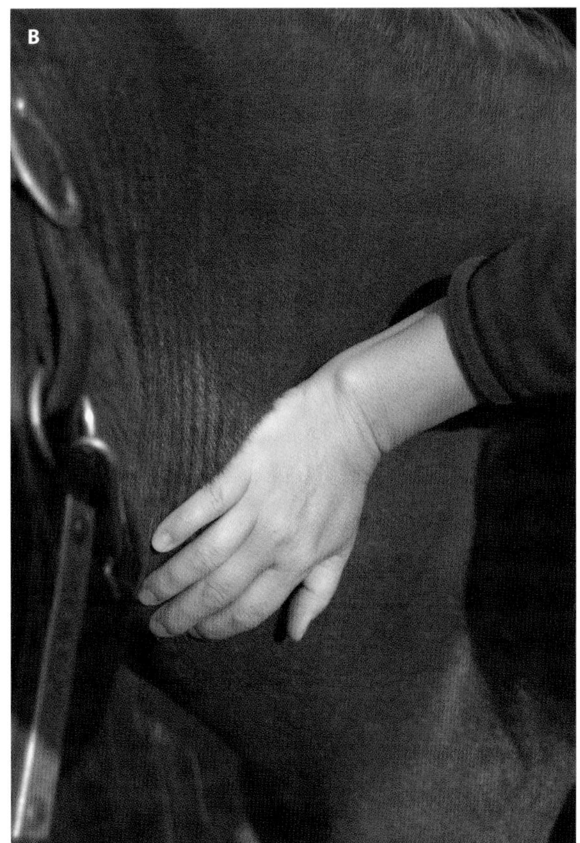

4.5 A & B Using the pisiform area of the hand, shown in A, is best for the neck Checkup. Note my elbow is pointed upward and my wrist is bent in B. This ensures the pressure from the hand is from the pisiform area.

BODY CHECKUP 5
THE C7
(7th Cervical Vertebra)

The 7th cervical vertebra (C7) is located underneath the shoulder blade. A subluxated C7 can cause numerous problems that are often blamed on something else. One helpful diagnostic is a basic forward shoulder stretch. In this stretch, you lift the horse's leg up and bring it forward: Stand in front of the horse, facing him with your hand holding his leg behind the knee. Stretch the leg forward, slowly lowering it toward the ground, and sliding your hand down to hold the leg behind the fetlock, while watching the shoulder (figs. 5.1 A–C).

Horses with C7, shoulder, shoulder blade (scapula), or (more uncommonly) front-rib subluxa-

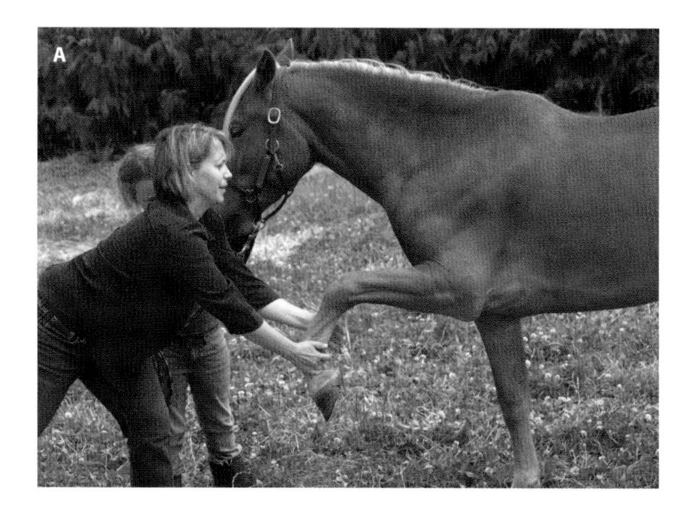

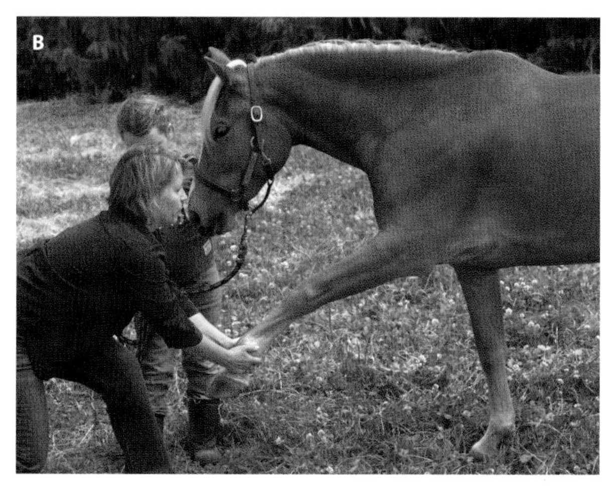

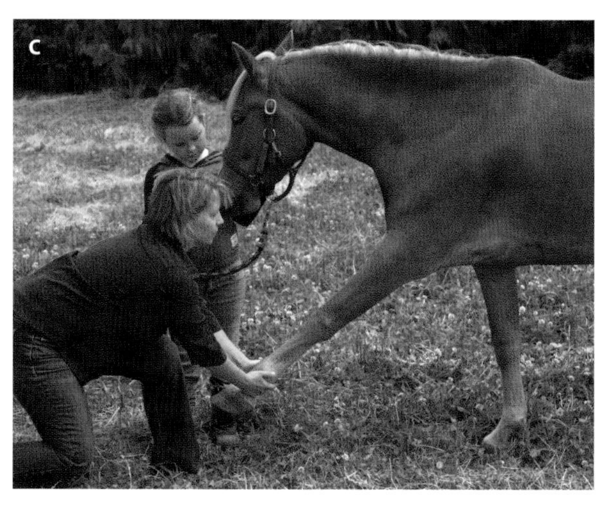

5.1 A–C This mare is showing a very good "fake" shoulder stretch. In A, the first clue that there is a problem is her uncomfortable expression when her leg starts to be pulled forward. In B, she looks comfortable enough with the leg stretch, but in C, as I try to get her to drop her leg and shoulder to the ground, she tenses up the shoulder-area muscles—I can't get the leg any further down to the ground than shown in the picture.

C7 CHALLENGE LEVEL ☆☆☆☆
Locating Anatomic Area: ☆☆☆☆
Positioning of Person or Horse: ☆☆☆
Subtle Range of Motion: ☆☆☆
Complex Evaluation of Checkup: ☆☆☆

tions will "fake" this stretch. They lower the leg down to the ground, but as you watch the shoulder, you will see that it does not move. Often a good massage can release the shoulder and shoulder-blade muscles enough to allow this stretch. However, if the horse has been worked on and has relaxed shoulder and shoulder-blade muscles, but continues to fake the stretch, you most likely are dealing with a C7 or shoulder subluxation.

Common Symptoms

BEHAVIORAL OR PERFORMANCE SYMPTOMS

Very Common

- Dropping the shoulder, especially around turns
- Going wide on turns

Frequent

- Holding the shoulder out wide on turns
- Short-striding in front
- Unable to do "long-and-low" work
- Lack of extension and/or ability to stretch in the front end
- Stiff in the front end
- Shoulder or shoulder blade have decreased range of motion

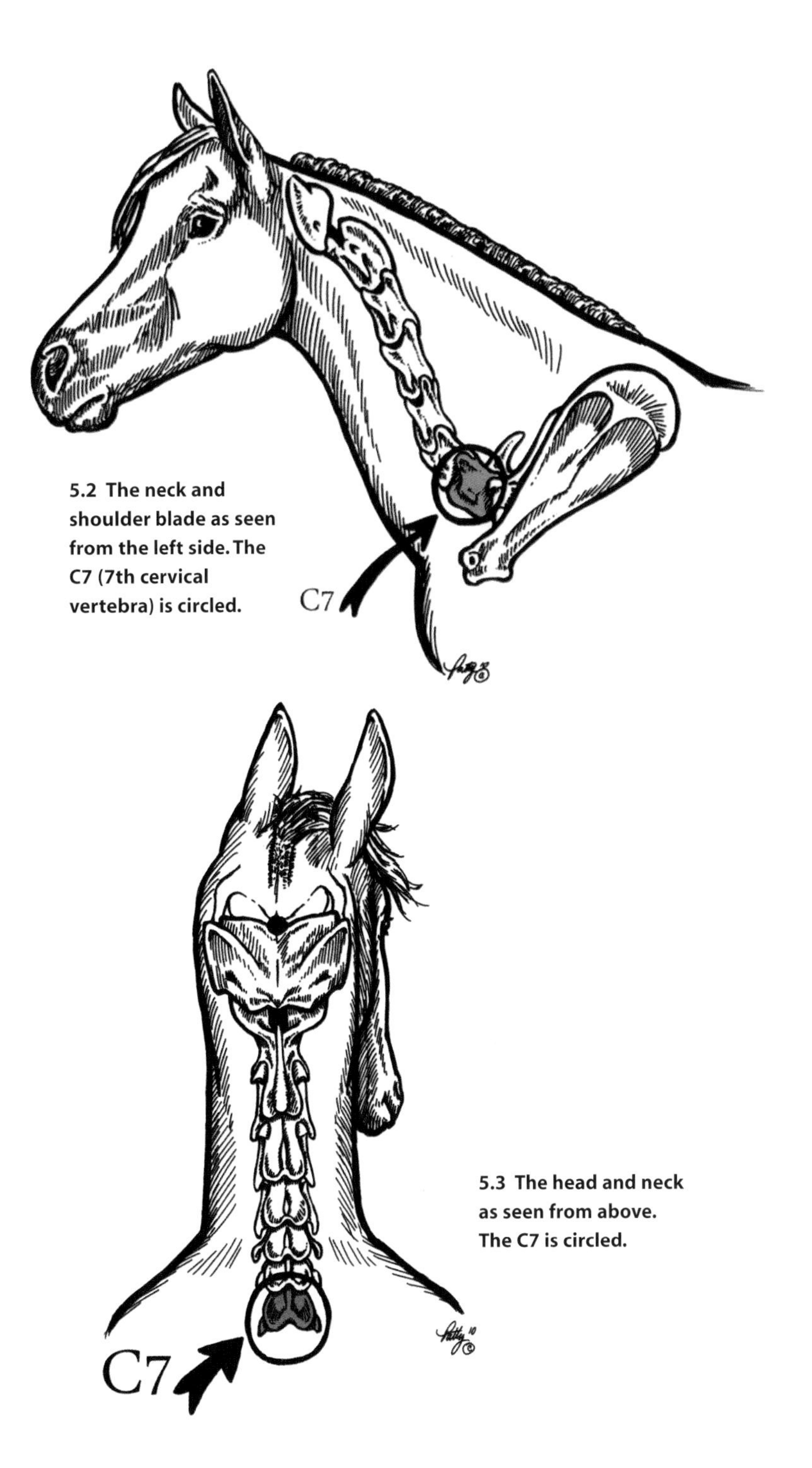

5.2 The neck and shoulder blade as seen from the left side. The C7 (7th cervical vertebra) is circled.

5.3 The head and neck as seen from above. The C7 is circled.

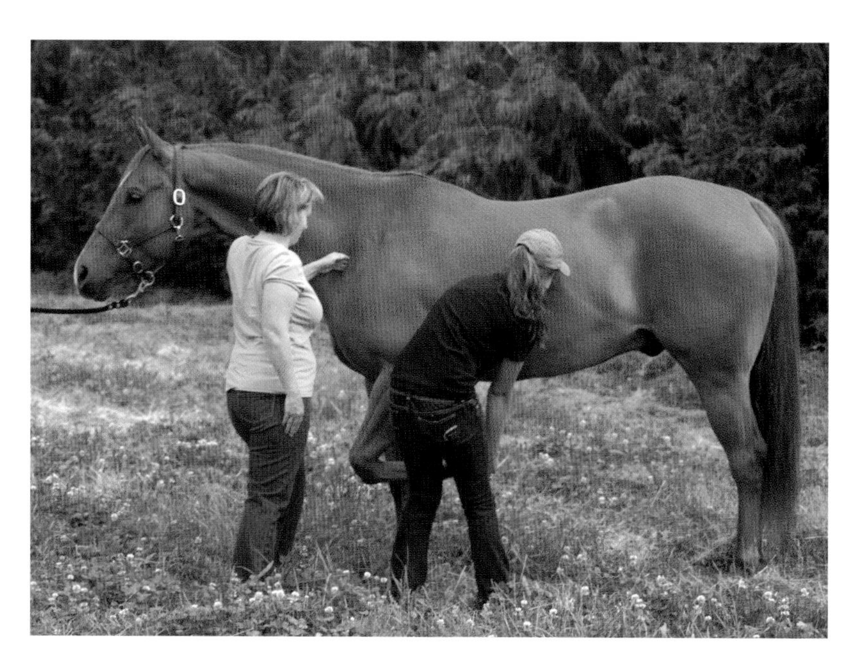

5.4 It's helpful to have a helper hold up the horse's leg for the C7 Checkup.

- Shoulder or shoulder blade is difficult to stretch

Occasional

- Stiff neck
- "Girthy"/"cinchy"
- Landing toe-first on front feet
- Tripping
- Sore shoulder-area muscles
- "Phantom" lameness in the front end

PHYSICAL SYMPTOMS: CURRENT OR PRIOR

- Shoulder, anything "weird" with it: "moving funny"
- Rib subluxations, recurrent
- Sternum subluxation
- "Clubby" foot
- Low-heel/ high-heel syndrome, tendency toward
- Ewe neck
- Withers, tight

Checkup Directions

FUNCTION: The C7 is the last vertebra in the neck (cervical spine). It lies underneath the shoulder blade (scapula) and is difficult to access. A C7 subluxation can cause numerous problems, yet the structures around the C7 are usually "blamed" for a problem as they are more prominent and easier to feel.

RANGE OF MOTION: The C7 technically has the same range of motion as the rest of the neck vertebrae. However, the C7 is "covered" by the shoulder blade. When moving, the horse lifts the shoulder out of the way to allow C7 to move through its entire range of motion. When standing, however, you are unable to check the entire range of motion and can usually only reach the part of the C7 that is closest to the neck instead of the entire vertebra. So you are feeling for some movement versus no movement at all, which (as mentioned before) feels like pushing on a solid, immoveable rock.

HOW TO

Stand at the horse's shoulder and face his rear end. The C7 is easier to check when you have someone lifting up the foot and making sure the horse's leg is relaxed (fig. 5.4). Otherwise, you must hold up the leg

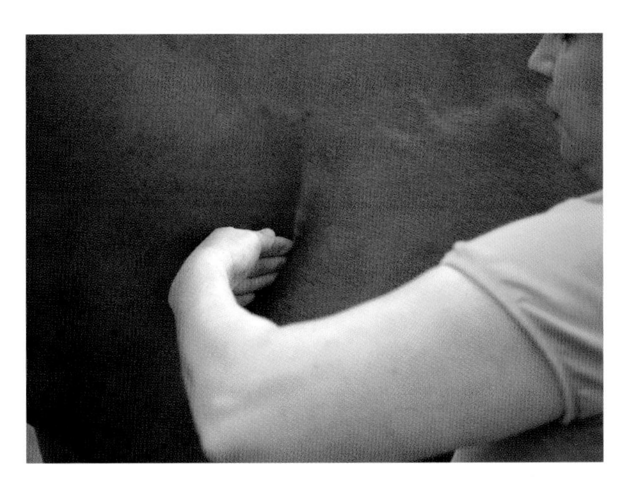

5.5 Slide your fingers under the cartilage cap at about the middle of the shoulder blade.

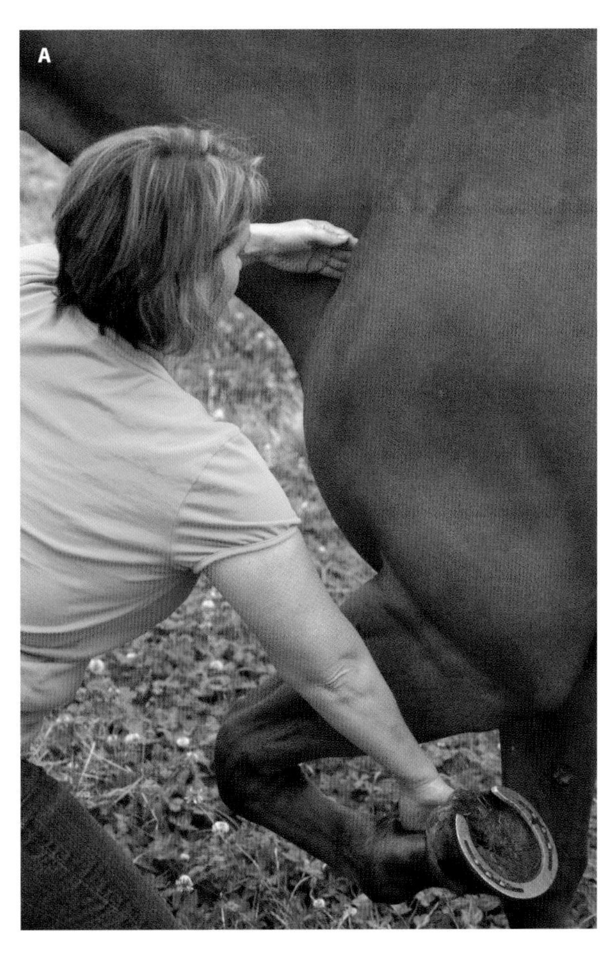

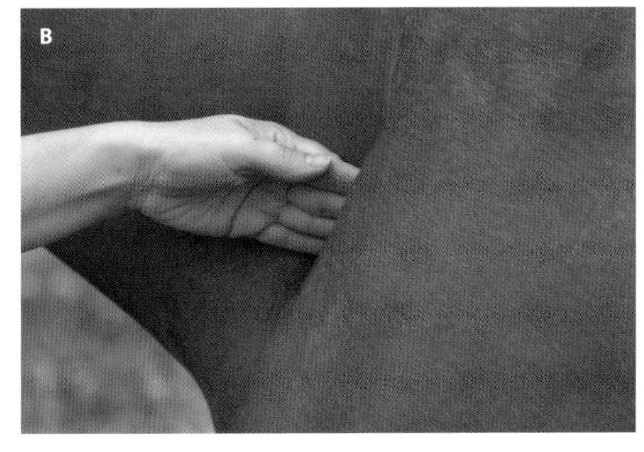

5.6 A & B Slide your hand down the shoulder blade until you can feel C7. Note in photo A I am standing out and to the side to allow the photo to be taken. It is easier when standing close in the horse, as seen in photo 5.7 on p. 64.

with one hand while performing the Checkup with the other. Once the horse becomes accustomed to having the C7 checked, it becomes much easier.

Slide your fingers (extended outward) under the "cartilage cap" at approximately the middle of the shoulder blade (fig. 5.5). Then slide your fingers down toward the ground until you can feel C7 (figs. 5.6 A & B). The C7 is the only large bone under there, approximately fist-sized. The ribs are past C7 (closer to the tail) and smaller.

Once you have found C7, let your fingers curl in (fig. 5.7), and then "bounce" C7 inward, pushing with as much force as you would trying to smush a round, blown-up balloon in half.

Diagnosis

If C7 seems to have a nice "give" or "bounce," and it feels the same on both sides of the horse, it is normal. Typically, a subluxated C7 will feel like an unmovable rock, or when C7 has subluxated to the side opposite of the side you are checking from, it may be hard to feel at all. So if you find the C7 vertebra difficult to locate, check it from the other side of the horse.

Another sign of a problem is when the horse is extremely reluctant to have your hand under his shoulder blade. In this case, the shoulder itself, or the ribs under it, may be subluxated, though it's possible that muscle stiffness or ligament tension may be holding the shoulder blade down. In this case a massage (or other modality such as acupuncture or laser therapy) may be needed to "release" the shoulder blade so you can get under it.

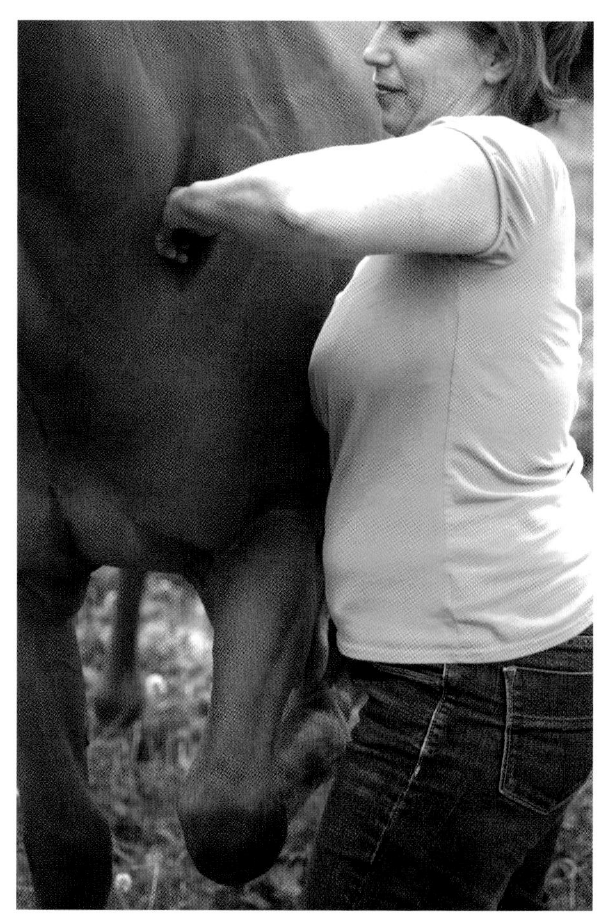

5.7 Note that my fingers have curled inward and I'm putting pressure on C7, pushing inward on the neck.

Summary: C7

- Any possible C7 subluxation, call chiropractor.
- No subluxation indicated, but symptoms remain, check for:
  - Chiropractic subluxations at: shoulder blade, shoulder, withers, ribs, sternum (pp. 66, 69, 108, 117, 74)
  - Saddle fit
  - Ulcers
  - TMJ or teeth issues
  - Navicular syndrome
  - Sore heels

Section 2

THE FRONT END BODY CHECKUPS

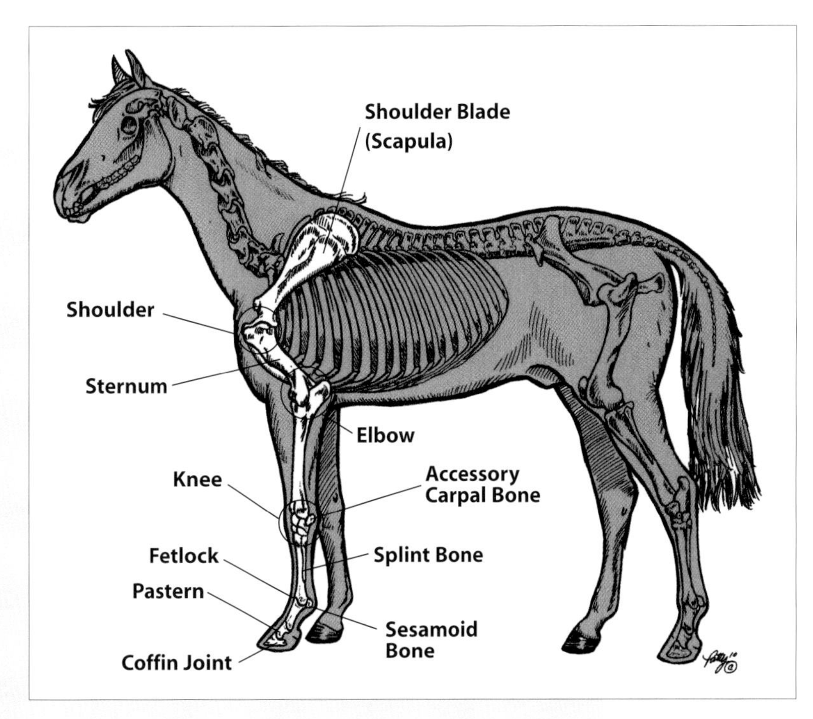

The Front End Body Checkup areas.

Front End Problems: General Symptoms

- Short-striding
- Stiff front leg(s) or shoulder(s)
- "Girthy"/"cinchy"
- Goes wide on turns
- Drops shoulder on turns
- Feels stiff in the front end
- Any shoulder difficulty
- Lack of forelimb extension
- Reluctance to stretch forelimb forward or backward
- Lameness or "offness" in front leg
- Tripping
- Reluctance to jump
- Stumbling on tight turns or around barrels
- Difficulty with front end lateral work
- Consistent interfering of front legs

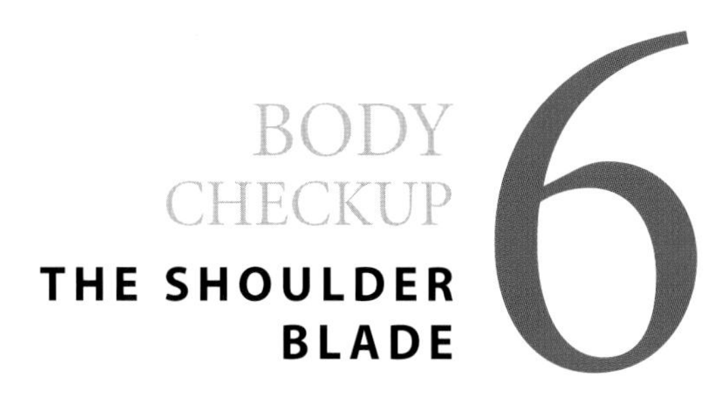

A 15-year-old Tennessee Walking Horse called Sweety was having difficulty bending at all to her left side. She had previously suffered a bad fall onto concrete and landed on that side. While adjusting her many chiropractic subluxations, I asked her owner if the shoulder blade muscle atrophy that was apparent had been gradual or if it had happened immediately after the fall.

Joyce, Sweety's owner, was shocked. "What atrophy? What is that? It sounds terrible!"

I had Joyce look at the shoulder-blade muscles and compare one side to the other. The left-side muscles were significantly smaller than the right. In fact, on the left side, the central edge of the scapula was very prominent, which is not normal.

This atrophy turned out to be reversible. It was due to subluxations causing the shoulder and shoulder blade to move in a manner that did not use the normal muscles, and after I adjusted Sweety, it was about 80 percent improved in a month. (Some cases of atrophy due to nerve damage, on the other hand, cannot be corrected.)

It's very easy to miss muscle asymmetries because we normally look at our horses from one side at a time. Periodically check your horse's muscles, comparing both sides for symmetry. Also check for hind-end muscle symmetry while looking at your horse from behind (be sure your horse is standing square for this). Don't forget to lift up the mane when you check the neck!

SHOULDER BLADE CHALLENGE LEVEL ☆☆☆
Locating Anatomic Area: ☆
Positioning of Person or Horse: ☆☆☆
Subtle Range of Motion: ☆☆
Complex Evaluation of Checkup: ☆☆☆

Common Symptoms

BEHAVIORAL OR PERFORMANCE ISSUES

Very Common

- Stiff front leg(s) or shoulder(s)
- Lack of front-end extension
- Decreased range of motion of shoulder or shoulder blade
- Reluctance to stretch front leg(s)

Frequent

- Goes wide on turns
- Anything "weird" with the shoulder
- Struggles with front-end lateral work

Occasional

- Short-striding
- "Girthy"/"cinchy"
- Drops shoulder on turns
- Tripping
- Interferes in front end
- Shoulder muscles, sore

PHYSICAL SYMPTOMS: CURRENT OR PRIOR

- Withers, one side higher than the other
- Low-heel/high-heel syndrome
- Wither subluxations, chronic
- Saddle, history of improper fit or difficulty fitting
- Rider feels crooked or saddle slips to one side

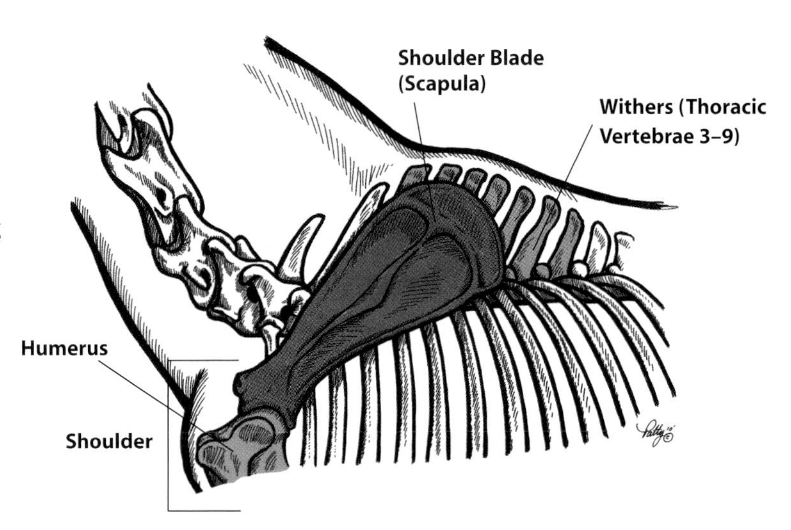

6.1 The left shoulder and withers area, as seen from the side.

Checkup Directions

FUNCTION: Because there is no bone-to-bone connection, the shoulder blade functions as the connection between the horse's body and the front leg with a "cartilage cap" around the margin of the shoulder blade, along with numerous muscles and fascia.

RANGE OF MOTION: Because the shoulder blade is only attached to the body via muscles and ligaments, it has quite a large range of motion. It should be able to move *at least* 2 inches up and down (4 inches is commonly seen), and 1 to 2 inches forward toward the head and backward toward the tail.

HOW TO

For this Checkup, lift the shoulder blade from its neutral standing position and evaluate how far you can move it. It should move easily and fluidly in all directions. The tricky part is to get your own body mechanics and hand positioning correct in order to isolate the shoulder-blade movement, eliminating as much shoulder movement as possible.

Lift the leg off the ground into a relaxed position. Cross your arms at the forearm level so you can comfortably hold the cannon bone with both hands. Be sure not to squeeze the tendons at the back of the leg. Step in toward the horse with your legs apart so

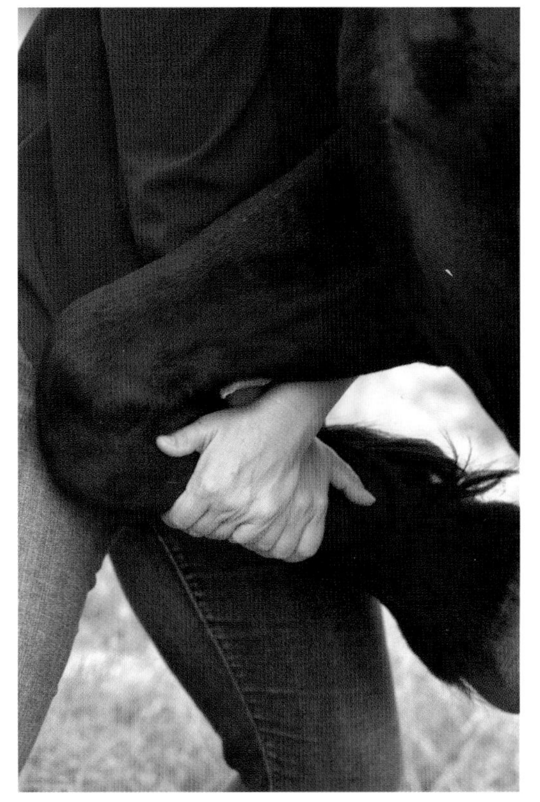

6.2 My arms are crossed so I can lift the horse's leg easily. I am careful not to squeeze the tendons along the back of the cannon bone. Note how I have stepped in close to the horse's body.

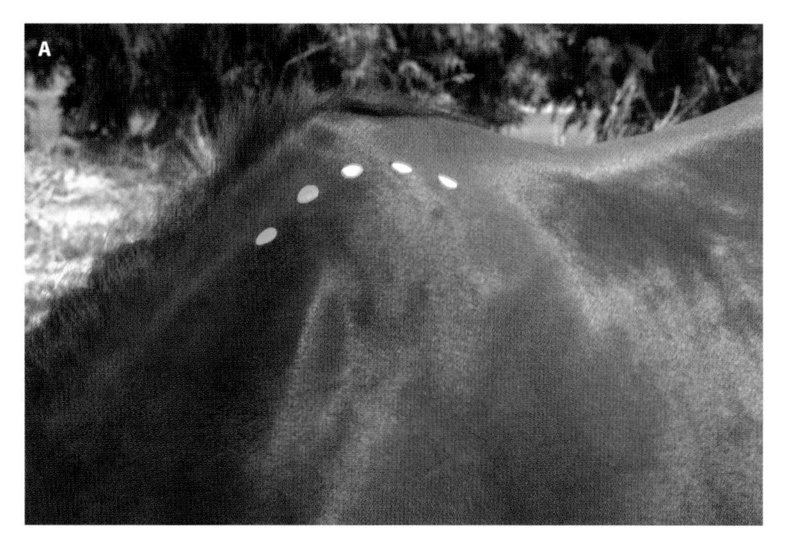

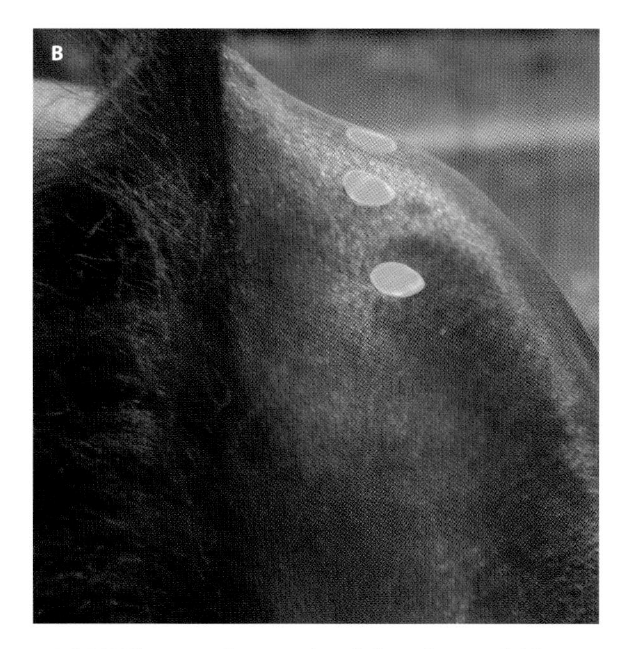

6.3 A & B The green dots are placed along the top of this horse's shoulder blade—you can see it here from two different angles. This is the area that you watch for movement upward during the Checkup. NOTE: Your horse's shoulder blades may be closer to, or further away from, the withers than seen on this horse.

that you can lift straight up. Your forearms should contact the horse's forearm (fig. 6.2). Now lift straight up and watch the top of the shoulder blade along the withers (figs. 6.3 A & B).

Diagnosis

The shoulder blade should move upward 2 to 4 inches, and it should move freely in all directions. If it does not, it is likely to be subluxated. Move the horse's leg forward and back. Be sure there is actually *shoulder-blade* movement—not just *shoulder* movement.

Generally speaking, a subluxated shoulder blade is the result of incorrect muscle tension caused by primary subluxations elsewhere. (An exception to this rule is trauma directly to the shoulder blade.) When other subluxations are corrected, the shoulder blade often will self-correct.

Summary: SHOULDER BLADE

- No shoulder-blade movement in any direction: Start with a good massage to relax the muscles. Often the shoulder blade will release once its muscles are relaxed. If it becomes "stuck" again a few days after the massage, it is subluxated. Call a certified chiropractor.
- No subluxation indicated but problems remain, check for:
  - Chiropractic subluxations at: shoulders, withers, ribs, sternum (pp. 69, 108, 117, 74)
  - Saddle fit
  - Heel-pain syndrome
  - Early flexor tendon strain
  - Hoof-wall imbalance

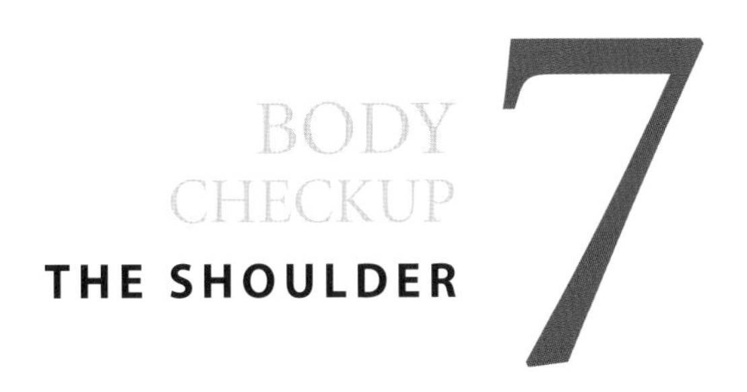

BODY CHECKUP 7
THE SHOULDER

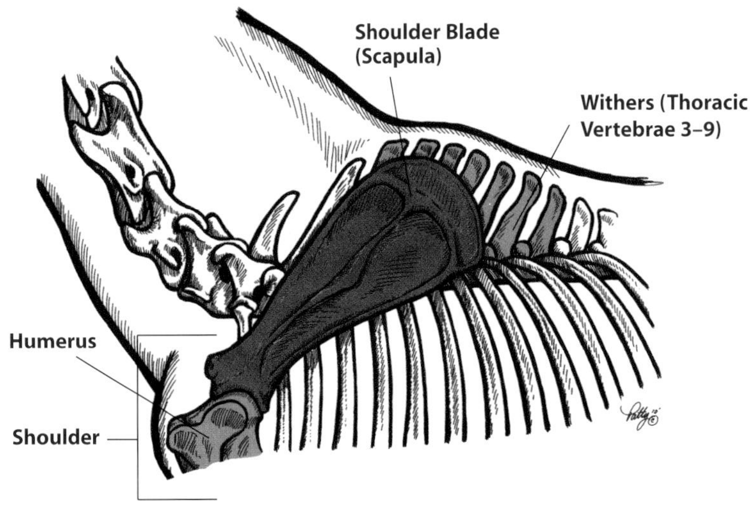

7.1 The left shoulder and withers area: side view.

When I was practicing traditional veterinary medicine, I received a number of panicked phone calls to the effect of, "Come quick! My horse's leg is broken. I think she got kicked in the shoulder."

Sure enough, the horse would be three-legged lame and barely able to walk back to the barn. This is very scary to see. However, nine times out of ten, the "broken leg" turns out to be a foot abscess.

The reason I mention this is that when anything is wrong in the front leg, most of the time it *looks* like it is in the shoulder. I believe this is because the shoulder is the area of greatest muscling in this part of the horse. When a horse moves his front leg abnormally for any reason, the shoulder muscle starts looking "funny."

If you think your horse has a shoulder problem, be sure to examine all the front leg structures, as well as the sternum, C7, withers, and ribs. Ribs that lie underneath the shoulder blade can also cause apparent shoulder problems. (The examination of these ribs is unfortunately beyond the scope of this book and you'll need to call a chiropractor with advanced certifications.)

Common Symptoms

BEHAVIOR OR PERFORMANCE SYMPTOMS

Very Common

- Any shoulder difficulty or "weirdness"
- Feels stiff in the front end
- Shoulder or shoulder blade decreased range of motion
- Tightness in shoulder or shoulder-blade movement
- Difficult to stretch shoulder
- Difficult to stretch front end
- Lack of extension in front end
- Goes wide on turns, possibly holds shoulder out

Frequent

- Struggles with front-end lateral work

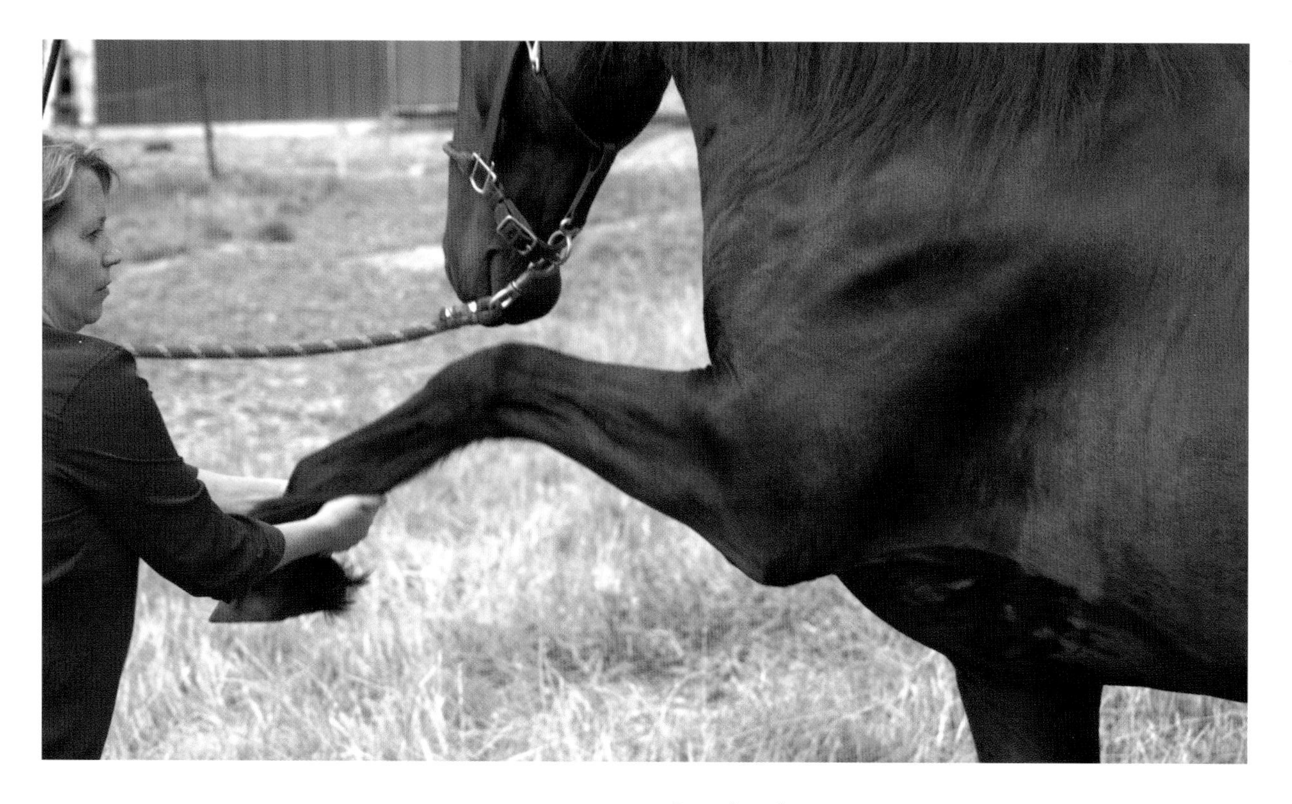

7.2 This photo was captured accidentally. I am not holding this mare's leg up at all—she stretched her leg up that far easily and gracefully (and probably because she was a bit bored). Notice how far up the horse's leg can reach, and how much shoulder—and shoulder-blade—muscling can be seen.

SHOULDER CHALLENGE LEVEL ☆☆☆
Locating Anatomic Area: ☆
Positioning of Person or Horse: ☆☆☆
Subtle Range of Motion: ☆☆
Complex Evaluation of Checkup: ☆☆☆

Occasional

- Short-striding in front, possibly only on turns
- Neck bending difficult, especially bending in front of the shoulder
- Drops shoulder on turns
- Shoulder muscles sore
- Interfering in front end

PHYSICAL SYMPTOMS: CURRENT OR PRIOR

- High shoulder (wither) on one side
- Low-heel/high-heel syndrome
- Rider feels crooked or saddle slips to one side
- Trouble with saddle fit

Checkup Directions

FUNCTION: The shoulder and shoulder blade are responsible for the majority of the movement control of the front leg.

NORMAL RANGE OF MOTION: The shoulder has quite a bit of movement available because the front leg is not attached to the rib cage (thorax) by any bones, only muscles (fig. 7.2). Because of this muscular attachment, there are three examinations to check shoulder movement.

HOW TO

TEST 1

Stand facing the horse's shoulder. Lift his front leg off the ground with one hand, and place your free hand just above the shoulder joint. Push directly back toward the tail. At a minimum, you should find at least 2 inches of movement toward the tail, and 4 or more inches of movement is very good (figs. 7.3 A & B).

TEST 2

Pick up the horse's front leg with both hands, and move the shoulder in a circle parallel to the ground (figs. 7.4 A & B).

TEST 3

Again grasp one front leg with both hands. Move the *shoulder in* toward the body while pulling the *elbow gently out.* Then push the elbow in while moving the shoulder out (fig. 7.5).

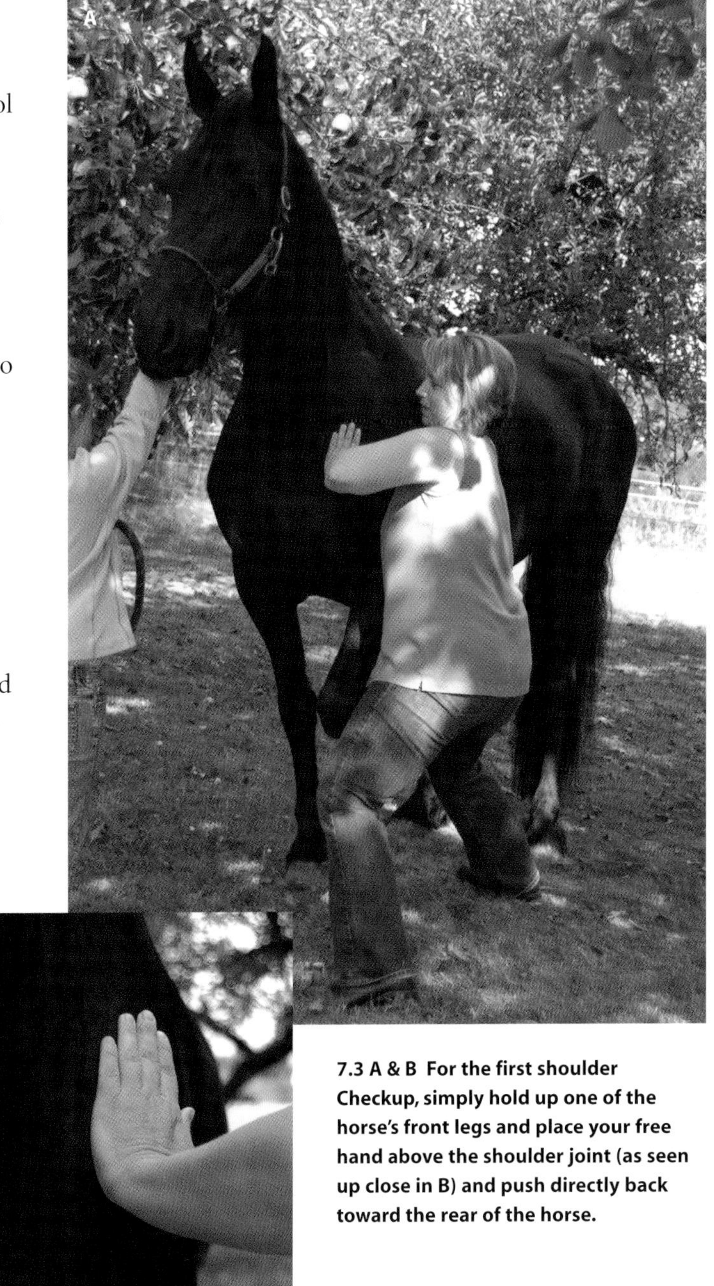

7.3 A & B For the first shoulder Checkup, simply hold up one of the horse's front legs and place your free hand above the shoulder joint (as seen up close in B) and push directly back toward the rear of the horse.

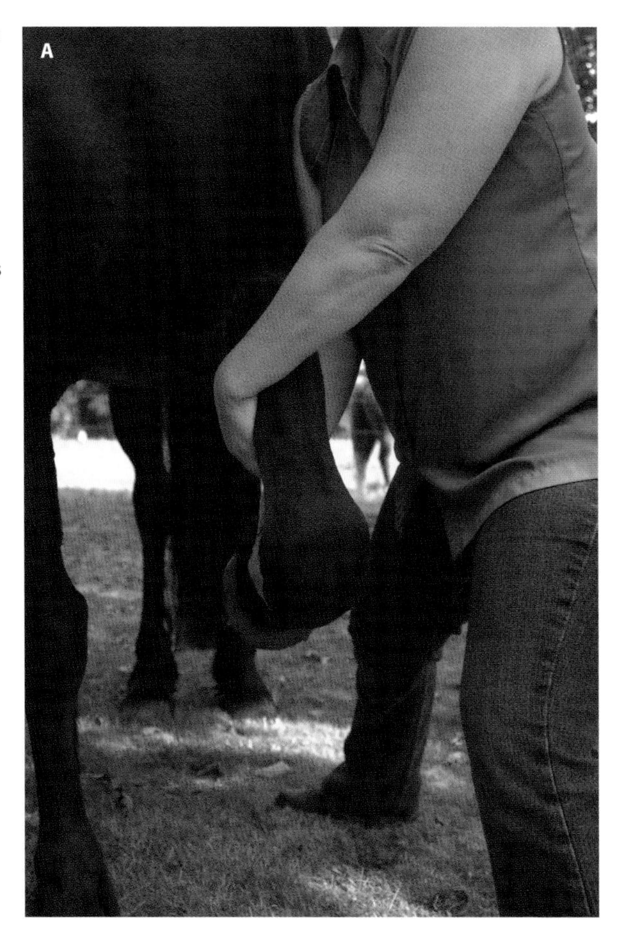

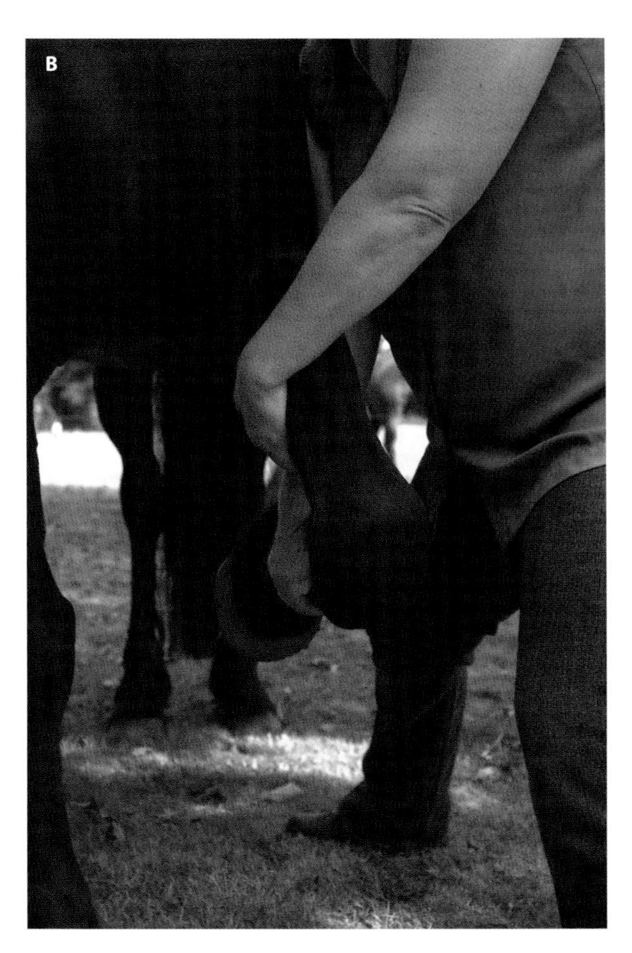

7.4 A & B Here you see two phases of the circular path that the shoulder should move through in Test 2. Note how I use my upper body to prevent the horse's shoulder blade from moving. (My hand position is more clearly shown in photo 7.5, p. 73.)

Diagnosis

TEST 1: When the shoulder can only be moved 2 inches or less back toward the tail, it may be subluxated. **TEST 2:** If there is a part of the circle that the shoulder is "reluctant" to be moved through, you have located a problem area. It could be caused by a subluxation, the shoulder joint itself may have an issue, or the shoulder muscles and tendons may be the primary problem. **TEST 3:** Again, if the shoulder is reluctant to move in or out from the body, it may be subluxated.

Summary: SHOULDER

▶ The shoulder Checkup, while not difficult to perform, can be difficult to interpret. This is because the tests move not only the shoulder, but also incorporate the shoulder blade and elbow. If either the C7, the sternum, or the withers are subluxated, shoulder movements may be hindered as a result. Nevertheless, when there is less movement than there should be, you have discovered a problem area that probably needs the help of the chiropractor.

And, if the muscles around the shoulder and shoulder blade are relaxed without tight areas, and the horse exhibits the "fake" shoulder stretch as described on p. 60 then the shoulder is probably subluxated. Your best bet is to have a chiropractor take a look at it.

▶ When symptoms remain with no signs of subluxation, check for:

- Chiropractic subluxations at: C7, shoulder blade, withers, sternum, ribs under shoulder (pp. 60, 66, 108, 74, 117)
- Shoulder bursitis (bicipital bursa inflammation)
- Heel-pain syndrome
- Saddle fit
- Early flexor tendon strain
- Hoof-wall imbalance

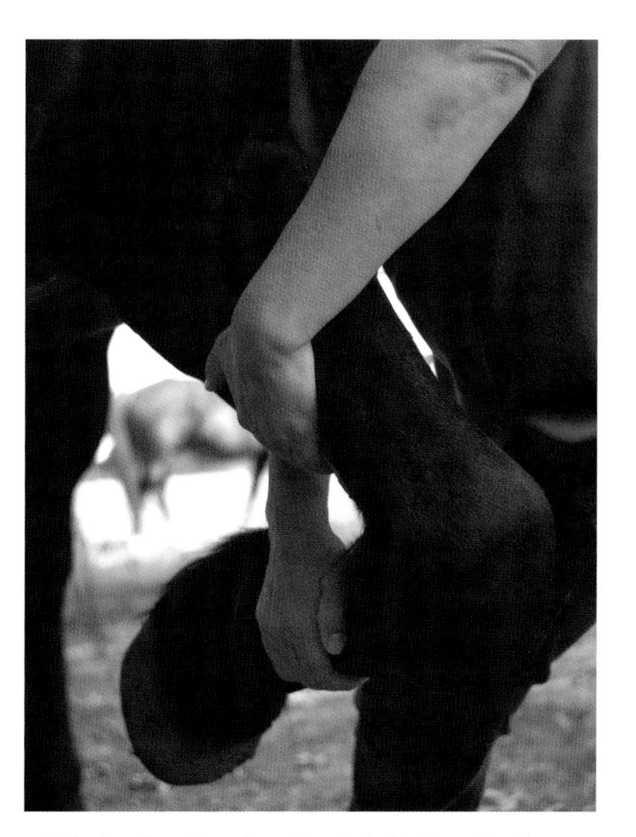

7.5 The hand position shown here is for both moving the shoulder in a circle (Test 2) and for Test 3, where I move the horse's shoulder and elbow in and out. In this photo, the elbow is in and the shoulder is pulled out.

BODY CHECKUP 8
THE STERNUM

I worked on a six-year-old Appaloosa mare named Bubbles whose new owner—Gail—used her for trail riding. Gail was very conscientious and concerned that Bubbles had trouble breathing, especially going downhill.

"Downhill?" I repeated. "Yes," Gail replied. "It's definitely worse downhill than uphill or on the flat. She acts like she's exhausted." I was surprised because it should be easier to breathe going downhill. (At least it is for me!)

Gail had had two vets check Bubbles' lungs. Bloodwork ruled out anemia and other possible problems. Everything looked normal.

At first, I found a lot of rib subluxations, which could explain breathing difficulties. But it didn't explain the downhill part of the mystery. As I continued to examine Bubbles, I found a small "dent" in her chest where some muscle was missing—apparently the result of a previous trauma.

It turned out that Bubbles' entire sternum was pushed back toward her tail, as well as to one side. This created a lot of tightness in her diaphragm, which attaches to the sternum, as she moved downhill.

Bubbles needed a few adjustments and some muscle work to keep her sternum in place, but after that she was immediately able to breathe normally when going downhill.

STERNUM CHALLENGE LEVEL ☆☆☆
Locating Anatomic Area: ☆☆
Positioning of Person or Horse: ☆☆
Subtle Range of Motion: ☆☆☆
Complex Evaluation of Checkup: ☆☆☆

Common Symptoms

BEHAVIORAL OR PERFORMANCE SYMPTOMS

*Very Common**

- Stiff, but may warm up to perform acceptably
- Difficulty bending in one or both directions

Frequent*

- Lack of front end extension
- "Girthy"/"cinchy"

Occasional

- Shortness of breath
- Exercise intolerance
- Interfering in front end
- "Phantom" lameness in front end
- Prefers to trot over other gaits

*(*It is rare for the sternum be subluxated alone. These very common and frequent symptoms typically occur when ribs are also subluxated.)*

PHYSICAL SYMPTOMS: CURRENT OR PRIOR

- Rider feels crooked or saddle slips to one side
- Rib subluxations that won't "correct" and/or are repeatedly "out"
- Lumbar subluxations, particularly one-sided
- Shoulder, shoulder blade, or C7 are difficult to "fix" and stay aligned
- Trouble with saddle fit

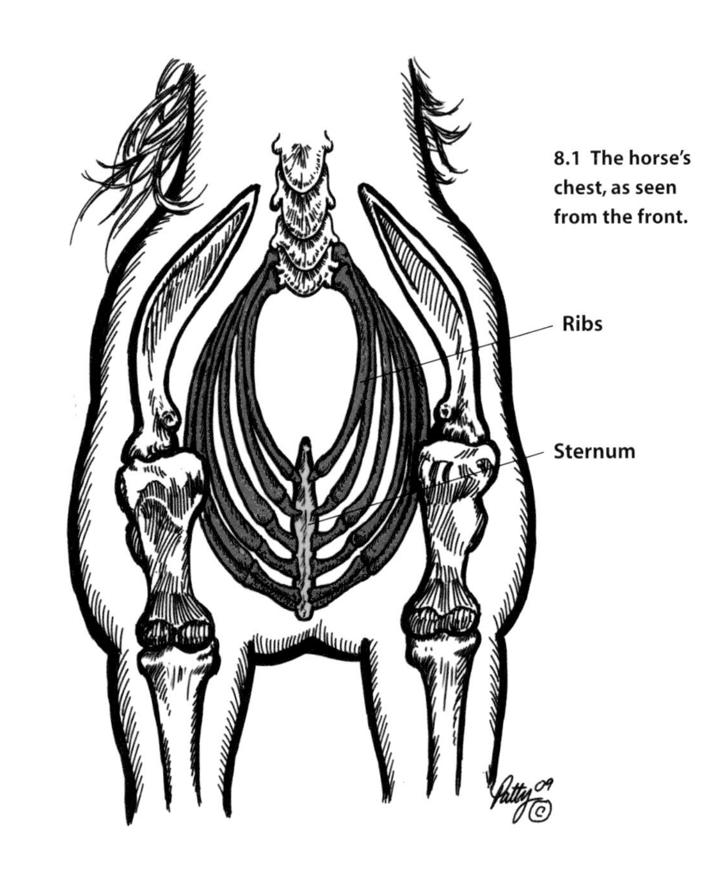

8.1 The horse's chest, as seen from the front.

Checkup Directions

FUNCTION: The first eight or nine ribs connect to the sternum. This provides a strong supporting structure for the chest. Because the chest of the horse does not attach to the front legs via bone (like the collar bone of the human), the sternum can be shifted over to one side as a result of traumatic force.

RANGE OF MOTION: Check the position of the sternum, not its official "range of motion." It does move forward and backward with lung expansion, but technically, the sternum does not have its own range of motion.

HOW TO

For this exam, the horse must stand absolutely square in front. Even one hoof, one-half inch off will change the muscle alignment and confuse the Checkup findings. Once the horse is standing square, locate the exact center of the sternal bone. This should be in the exact center of the chest (pectoral) muscles. You locate the center of the sternal bone by feeling for the edges of it. It is typically 3 to 5 inches wide (fig. 8.2). Bring your fingers in from the edges of the sternal bone to the center of the sternal bone, and check visually to determine the center of the chest muscles.

Diagnosis

The center of the sternal bone should be in the center of the chest muscles. When it is not, the sternum is subluxated. Check both the front of the sternum, located between the front legs, as well as the rear of the sternum, located a hands length behind the girth. Both areas need to be checked because the sternum can be subluxated only partially or at an angle.

Summary: STERNUM

- With evidence of subluxation in the sternum, call chiropractor.
- No subluxation found, check for:
  - Chiropractic subluxations of: ribs under shoulder, withers, shoulder (pp. 117, 108, 69)
  - Saddle fit
  - Ulcers
  - Barrel, "rolled" (rare and requires a structural integration professional—Rolfing or Hellerwork—to correct it)

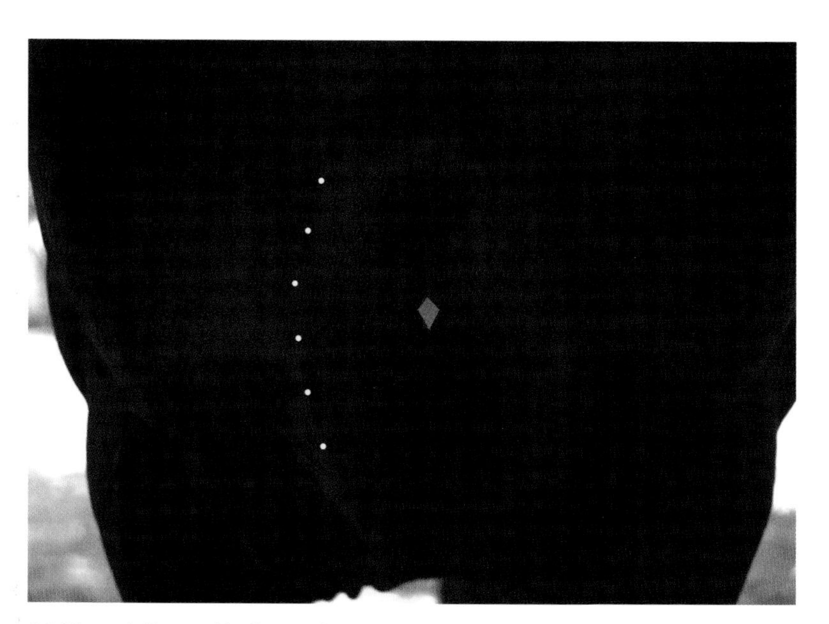

8.2 The red diamond indicates the center of the sternum. The white dots delineate the edges of the sternal bone.

BODY CHECKUP 9

THE ELBOW

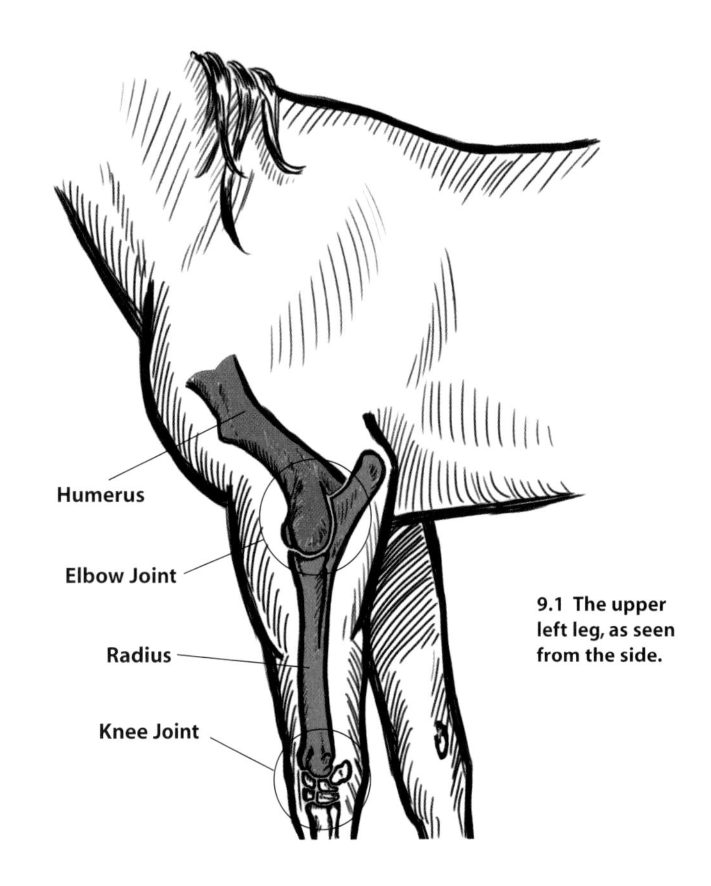

9.1 The upper left leg, as seen from the side.

Rico was a miniature donkey. No one knew how old he was. But he was very sweet and loved to have his long, velvety ears rubbed. So he stayed around the farm. He loved to stand under the horses whenever it rained.

Rico had quite the trouble with a sole abscess in his left front foot. Because donkey hoof walls are so tough, abscesses can be tricky to get out. He had been soaked in Epsom salts and wrapped for over a month. Nancy, his owner, was getting quite tired of it.

She informed me that she thought she saw "the 'goopi-di-goo' come out along his coronary band" a few weeks back. After that the heat was gone from his hoof. "But he is still just about as 'crickity,'" she said. "It is quite the puzzlement." (I love her vocabulary. I try to use her words whenever I can.)

I checked out Rico's body first—before his legs—because I didn't have to kneel down on the ground to do so. While doing so (and not finding much wrong), I asked Nancy more questions. "Has he been doing anything weird?" I asked. "I mean weird for Rico?" I qualified.

Nancy replied that the only different thing he had been doing was putting his foot in the water trough to try and get the wrap off. He usually succeeded by the end of the day. But since she took off the wrap twice a day anyway, she didn't try to stop Rico from his "good natured shenanigans."

This revelation narrowed it down for me. Once I adjusted his elbow, shoulder, and shoulder blade, Rico was moving quite nicely. A few more weeks of rest without the wrap "shenanigans," and Rico was back to his old donkey self.

Common Symptoms

BEHAVIORAL OR PERFORMANCE SYMPTOMS

Very Common

- Lack of forelimb extension
- Short-striding, or "off" in front, possibly turns only

Frequent

- Reluctance to stretch forelimb forward or backward
- Decreased range of motion in shoulder
- Tight movement in shoulder
- Reluctance to stretch shoulder

Occasional

- Trouble with front-end lateral work
- Interfering in the front end
- Foot landing toe first
- Tripping regularly

PHYSICAL SYMPTOMS: CURRENT OR PRIOR

- Leg "hits the ground heavy"
- Other leg joints have history of subluxations or injury
- Shoulder-area tightness

ELBOW CHALLENGE LEVEL ☆☆☆☆
Locating Anatomic Area: ☆
Positioning of Person or Horse: ☆☆
Subtle Range of Motion: ☆☆☆☆
Complex Evaluation of Checkup: ☆☆☆☆

- Foot, problems with "club" foot, or tendency to grow excess heel
- Foot, problems with medial-lateral hoof wall imbalance
- Knee, "bobbing" or "buckling over"

Checkup Directions

FUNCTION: The elbow's function is to assist in the transfer of ground forces and forelimb extension.

RANGE OF MOTION: The horse's elbow joint is anatomically very similar to a human's. While the majority of the elbow joint's movement occurs in the flexor-extension pathway, this is not when subluxations typically occur. It is much more common for the elbow to be subluxated in its side-to-side movement. The side-to-side range of motion can be small (approximately one-half to 1 inch) in horses that hold their legs tight to their body. It can also be larger (approximately 1 to 3 inches) in horses with big, relaxed joints. Therefore, evaluation of this Checkup can be tricky.

HOW TO

For this Checkup, hold the horse's leg off the ground; it should be relaxed. When checking the left leg, hold the leg up with your left hand at the mid-cannon bone area. This hand will keep the rest of the leg still while the other hand moves the elbow.

Place your free hand just below the elbow joint—this is directly below the point of the elbow (figs. 9.2 A & B). If you place your hand directly on the joint you are evaluating, your hand will impede the movement, no matter how lightly you touch.

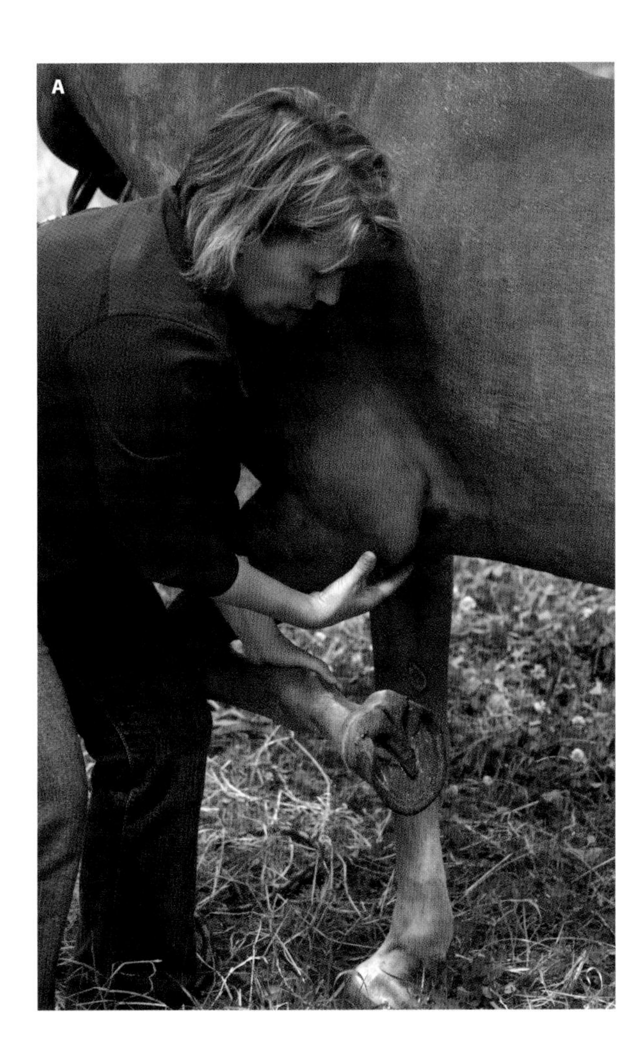

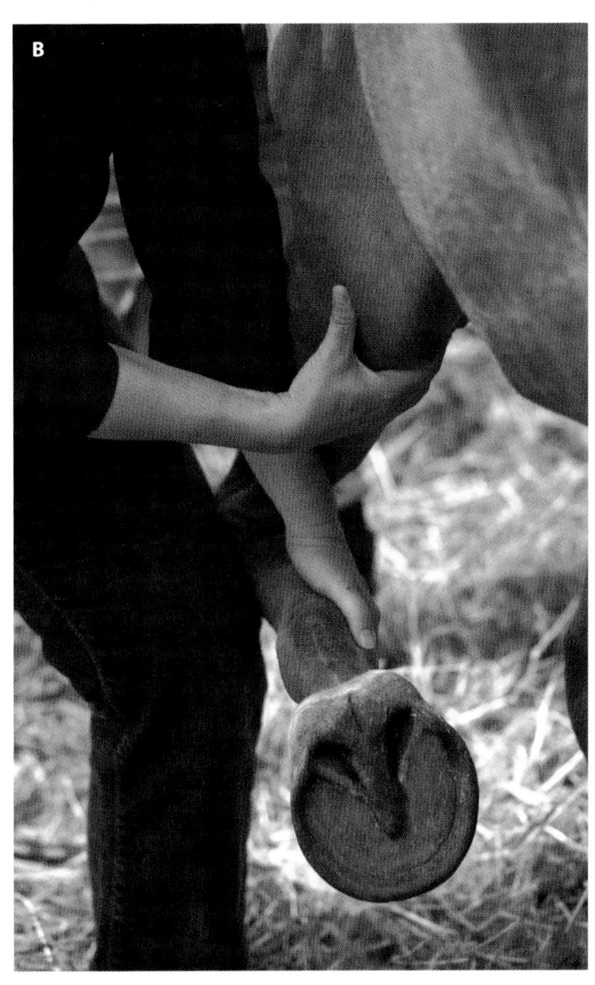

9.2 A & B Here I demonstrate the correct position for the elbow Checkup. Note in photo B the use of my forearm and knee to prevent the rest of the horse's leg from moving while the elbow is checked.

With the leg still held off the ground and relaxed, pull the elbow toward you, then push the elbow in toward the body. The movement of the elbow in and out includes both the elbow joint's side-to-side movement as well as a little bit of shoulder and shoulder-blade movement (figs. 9.3 A–C).

Diagnosis

When the elbow joint is subluxated, it is often fairly obvious. The elbow's movement in one direction (toward or away from the body) is noticeably stiff, stuck, and/or the horse won't allow the movement. Look for the range of motion of the elbows to be the same on both front legs. Asymmetry between legs usually indicates subluxation.

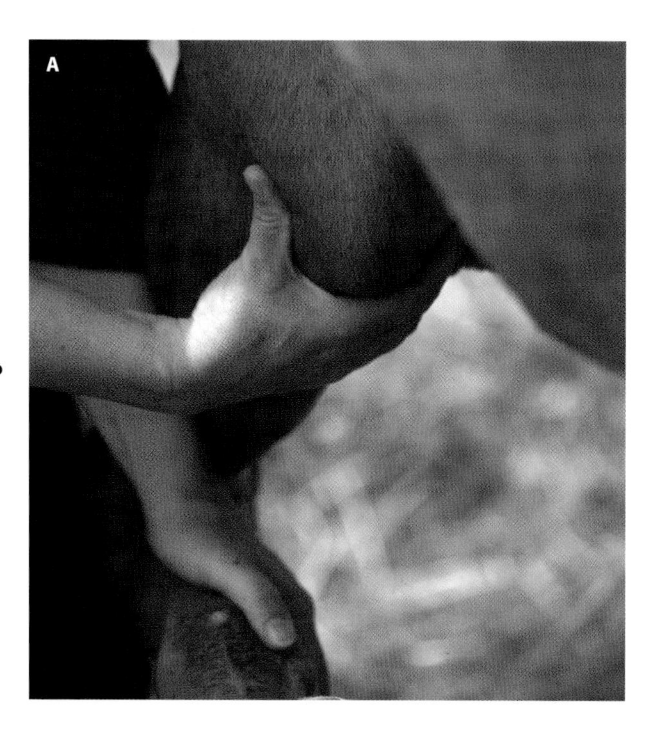

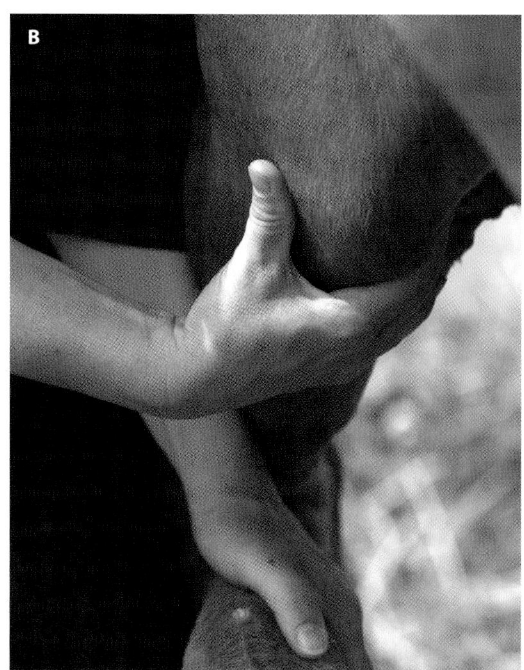

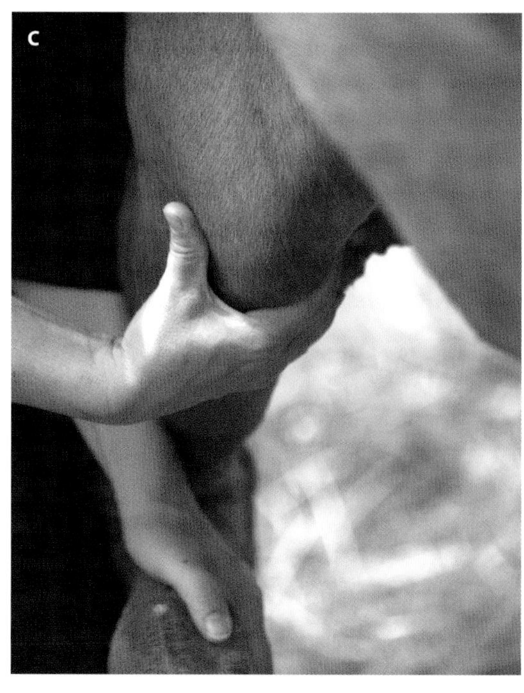

9.3 A–C Here you can see the movement of the left elbow. In A, the elbow is closest to the horse's body, B shows the middle position, and C shows the elbow furthest away from the body. This is a subtle movement to both see and feel.

NOTE: It is unusual for the elbow joint to be the primary chiropractic problem, so be sure to do your shoulder and shoulder blade (scapula) Checkups (pp. 69 and 66).

Summary: ELBOW

- When subluxation indicated, call chiropractor.
- No subluxation found, however symptoms remain, check for:
  - Subluxations at: shoulder, shoulder blade (scapula), C7, knee (pp. 69, 66, 60, 81)
  - Hoof-wall imbalance
  - Navicular syndrome
  - Sore heels
  - Coffin joint issues in opposite front leg

BODY CHECKUP 10
THE KNEE

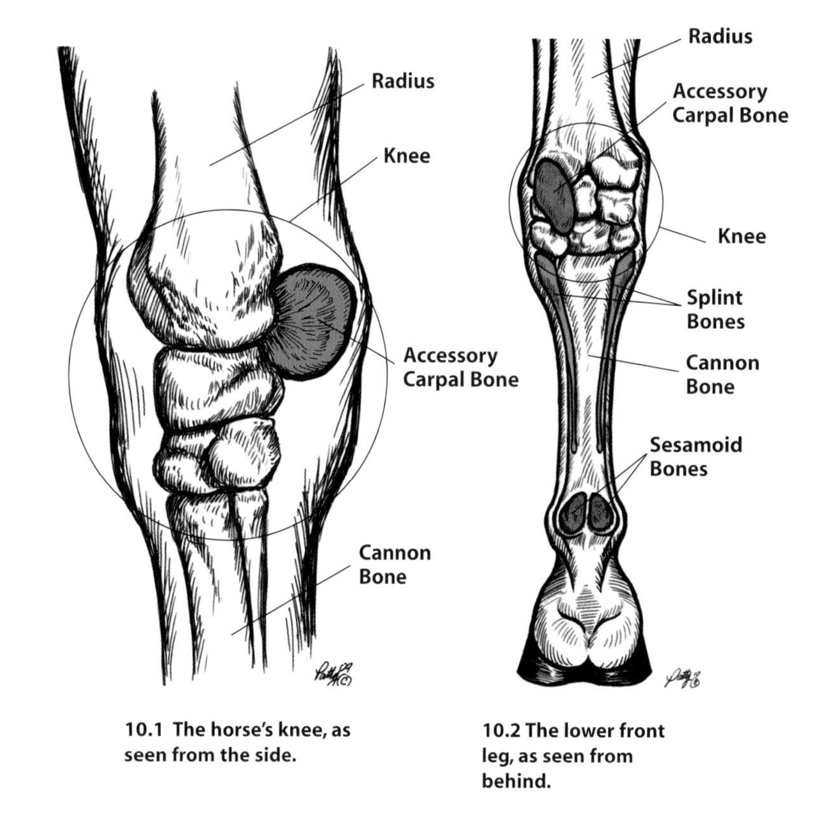

10.1 The horse's knee, as seen from the side.

10.2 The lower front leg, as seen from behind.

Damsel is a lovely Andalusian mare, 12 years of age. Her owner, Diane, wanted me to look Damsel over because she was thinking of breeding her. Her concern was that she was "over at the knee." This term refers to the top of the knee "protruding" over the bottom of the knee, especially when viewed from the side. It is considered a conformational fault and something you wouldn't want in a broodmare.

Looking over each knee from the side, I noted that she was indeed over at the knee, but only mildly.

"Diane," I said, "I really don't think it's a problem. I want you to take a picture with your phone of this problem. Make it the worst picture you can."

"Are you crazy?" she asked.

"No," I replied. "I am not crazy. Not today, at least. I have an idea, and I'd like you to take a picture so that we know that neither of us is insane."

As I checked this mare out and adjusted her from head to toe, I found that both her shoulders and shoulder blades needed adjusting. I had wondered if that would be the case because her shoulder muscles looked suspiciously tight, particularly in the front part of the shoulders. Immediately after I finished her adjustment, Damsel took a few steps forward and reset her stance. Her knees were suddenly perfect! I was very pleased and Diane was running from side to side, getting lots of pictures the "new" knees.

And now I have let you in on a secret: Conformation is changeable.

Common Symptoms

BEHAVIORAL OR PERFORMANCE SYMPTOMS

Very Common

- Short-striding in front
- Tripping
- Decreased knee flexion

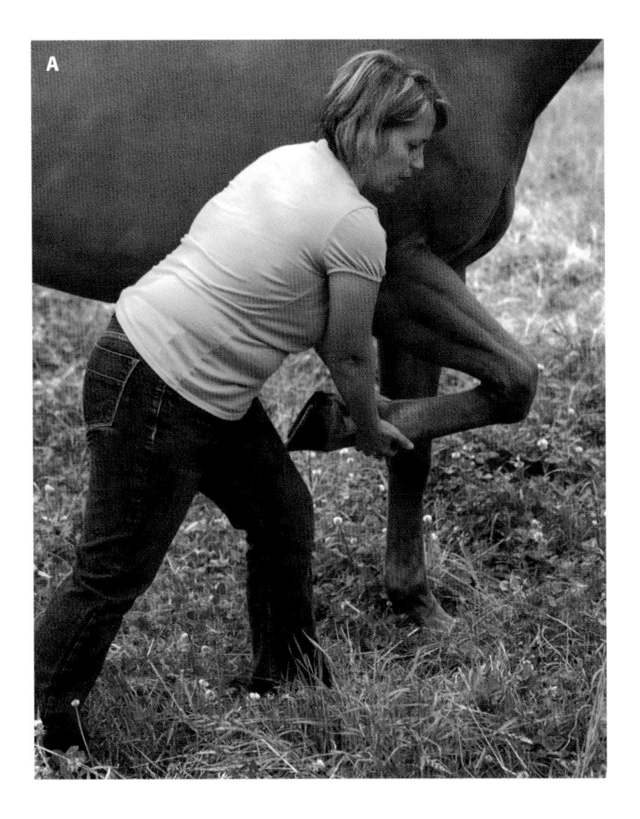

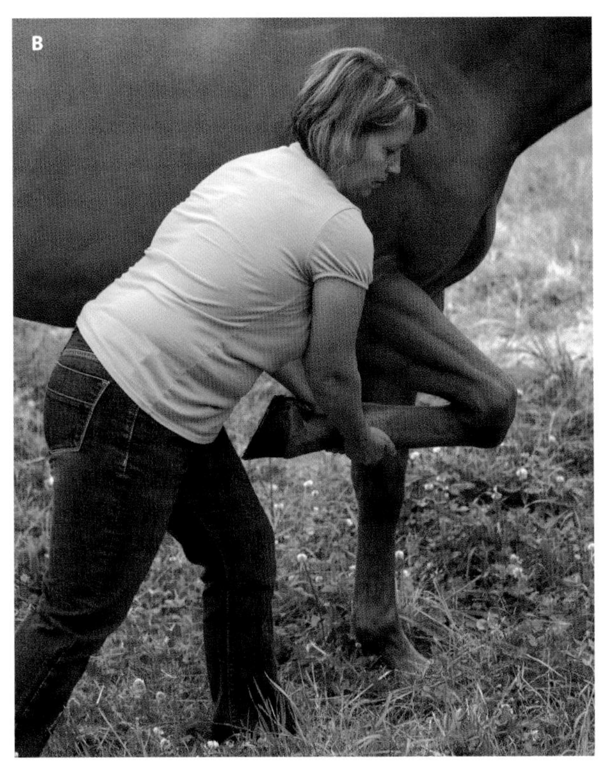

10.3 A–C In A, the horse is relaxed at the start of knee flexion, B shows partial flexion, and C shows complete knee flexion. Note there is no tension in the shoulder muscles, even with the knee completely flexed.

KNEE CHALLENGE LEVEL ☆
Locating Anatomic Area: ☆
Positioning of Person or Horse: ☆
Subtle Range of Motion: ☆
Complex Evaluation of Checkup: ☆

Frequent

- "Bobbing" or "buckling over" at the knee when standing
- Reluctance to jump

Occasional

- Lameness or "offness" in front leg
- Foot lands toe first
- Stiff in the front end
- Reluctance to stretch or extend in front end

PHYSICAL SYMPTOMS

- Foot "clubby" or tendency to grow excess heel

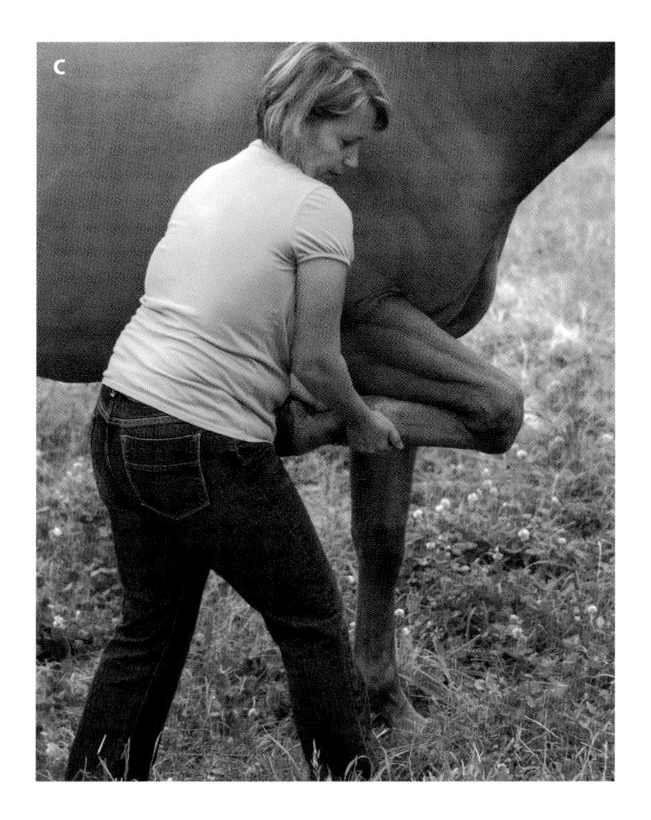

Checkup Directions

FUNCTION: The horse's knee (carpus) is anatomically very similar to the human wrist. In the horse, the knee is responsible for front leg flexion (i.e. bending at the knee).

The knee should not be confused with the stifle in the hind leg. It is easy to confuse these because the stifle looks like a human knee anatomically. But, officially, there is no "knee" in the horse's hind leg.

RANGE OF MOTION: The knee should be able to flex so that the cannon bone can touch the forearm (radius) with no resistance or discomfort anywhere in the front leg or shoulder area.

HOW TO

Lift the horse's leg with your hand under the fetlock or cannon bone and bend the knee until the horse tenses up, or until the cannon bone touches the forearm (figs. 10.3 A–C). Do not force the knee past the point of tension or resistance.

Diagnosis

When the bend is less than perfect—cannon to forearm—there may be a subluxation or arthritis involved. Check both knees and compare their range of motion. When they have the same range of motion, it is most likely *not* a chiropractic issue.

NOTE: Also check the accessory carpal bone of the knee (p. 84).

Summary: KNEE

- Less-than-perfect knee bend signifying probability of subluxation, call chiropractor.
- When Checkup is fine but common symptoms remain, check for:
    - Subluxations at: accessory carpal bone, shoulder, fetlock (pp. 84, 69, 90)
    - Knee arthritis
    - Hoof-wall imbalance
    - Hoof wall angles incorrect
    - "Joint mice" in knee
    - Tendons and ligaments tight due to mineral imbalance

BODY CHECKUP 11
THE ACCESSORY CARPAL BONE

Prophet was a three-year-old Quarter Horse destined to be a barrel racer. I was checking him to make sure he was ready to start in with some light training. So far, he had just been a "horse," hanging around the pasture and making a nuisance of himself.

As I checked him over, things went pretty well: Just a few minor rib and lumbar adjustments, certainly to be expected with a "youth" who liked to run up to fences and stop at the very last minute. Or, at least, try to stop—it was apparent there were a few times he hadn't completely stopped before the fence hit him in the chest. Then, when I was checking his right knee, it "popped," sounding just like someone popping their knuckles. And, it did it every time I flexed the knee.

I found a bone in Prophet's knee that needed adjustment, then I asked the horse's owner to walk him out for a minute to allow the adjustment to "take." But when I picked up the right foot again, it still popped.

I rechecked the entire front leg. I finally found that the accessory carpal bone was in need of help. Many of the important tendons of the leg, such as the superficial and deep digital flexor tendons, cross the accessory carpal bone as they come from above the knee to their position by the cannon bone.

After the accessory carpal bone was adjusted, Prophet's knee stopped its popping, and his owner could start thinking about winning her next barrel race.

ACCESSORY CARPAL BONE CHALLENGE LEVEL	☆☆☆
Locating Anatomic Area:	☆☆
Positioning of Person or Horse:	☆
Subtle Range of Motion:	☆☆☆
Complex Evaluation of Checkup:	☆☆

Common Symptoms

BEHAVIORAL OR PERFORMANCE SYMPTOMS

Very Common

- Decreased knee flexion

Occasional

- Short-striding in front, possibly on turns only
- Knee "bobbing" or "buckling over"

PHYSICAL SYMPTOMS: CURRENT OR PRIOR

- Knee or fetlock arthritis
- Leg hitting ground more heavily than the other legs (discernable by sound)
- Fetlock, decreased flexion
- Foot has medial-lateral hoof-wall imbalance
- Foot is "clubby" or tends to grow excess heel

Checkup Directions

FUNCTION: The accessory carpal bone is covered with tendon and ligament connections, both to the knee and to the leg. It helps distribute non-vertical forces throughout the knee and leg, and to facilitate rotation within the knee.

RANGE OF MOTION: The range of motion of the accessory carpal bone is small and subtle, very similar to the sesamoid bones (p. 94). It should be able to move freely in all directions approximately one-quarter inch.

HOW TO

The accessory carpal bone is located on the back of the knee, toward the outside (lateral side) of the leg (figs. 11.3 A & B). It is easier to feel it than to see it. Hold the knee up and then feel the back of the knee (fig. 11.4). The accessory carpal bone is the only "small lump" you can feel in this position.

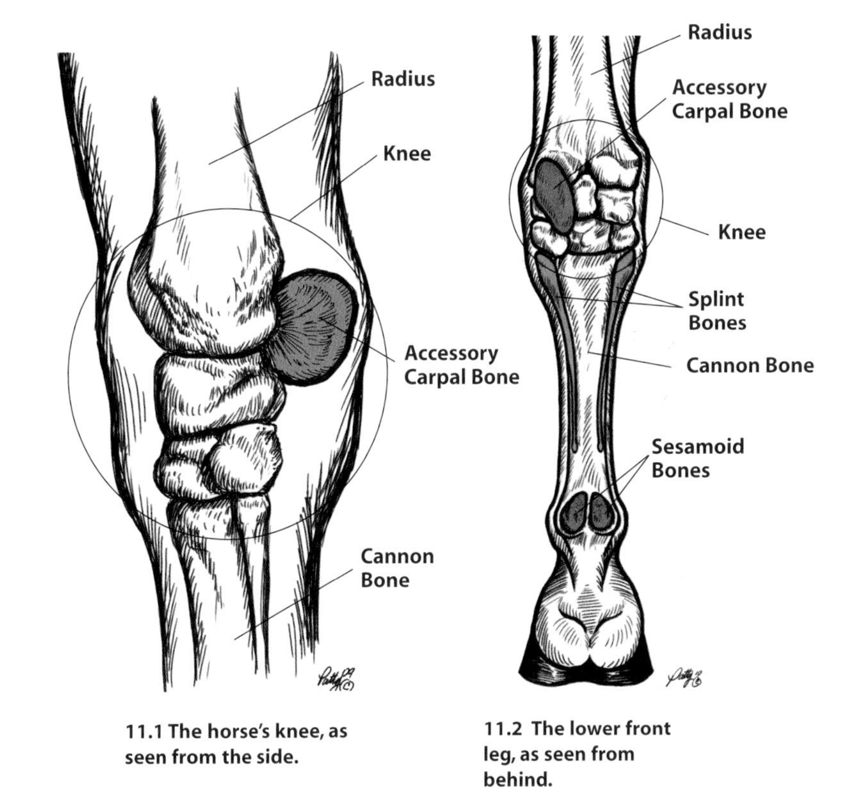

11.1 The horse's knee, as seen from the side.

11.2 The lower front leg, as seen from behind.

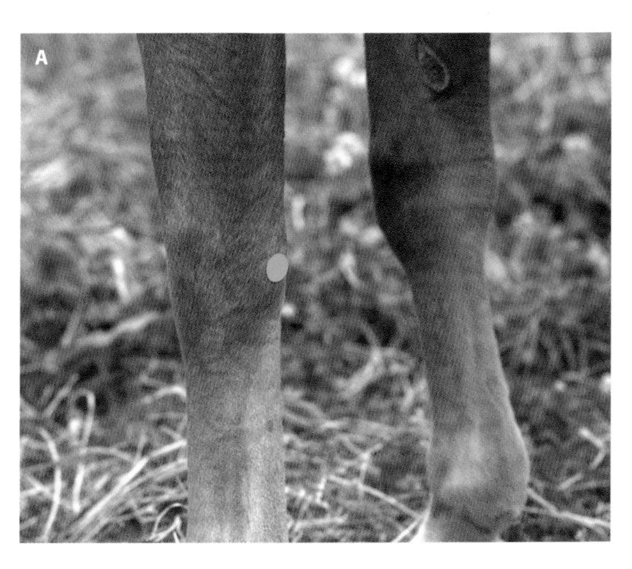

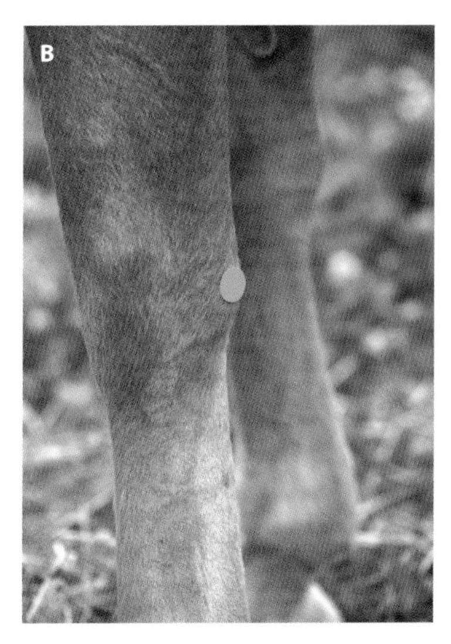

11.3 A & B The location of the accessory carpal bone, viewed from two different angles and marked by the green dot.

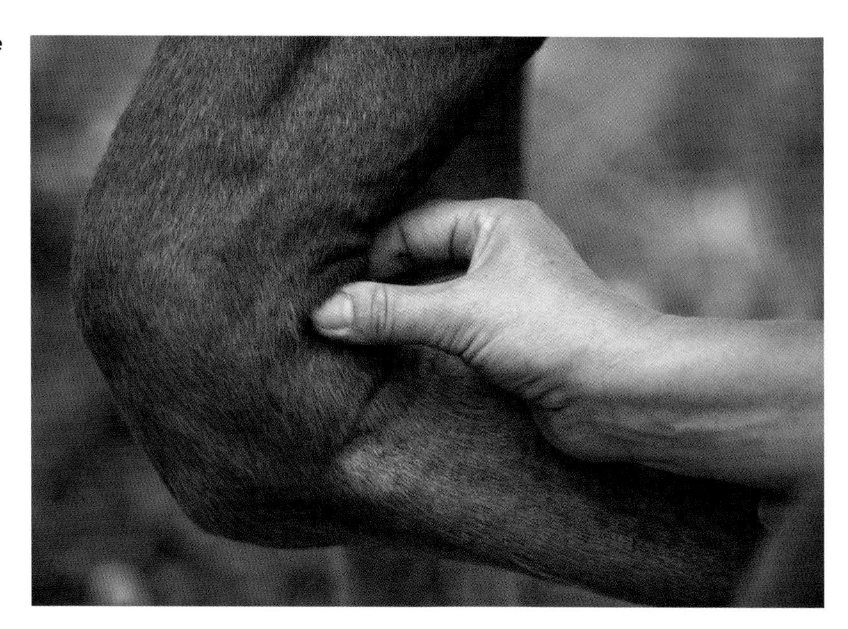

11.4 I demonstrate how to feel the accessory carpal bone.

Continuing with the horse's leg off the ground in a relaxed position, use gentle finger pressure to move the accessory carpal bone in all directions. It should be able to circle like a clock about one-quarter inch in all directions.

Diagnosis

If there is no movement—or less movement—in one direction as compared to the others, you most likely have a subluxation of the accessory carpal bone. But, if the bone doesn't seem to move much at all, especially as compared to the other leg, the horse may have arthritis or a vitamin or mineral imbalance affecting the tendons and ligaments (see p. 19).

Summary: ACCESSORY CARPAL BONE

▶ Because the accessory carpal bone is covered with tendons and ligaments, it is important to make sure your horse is consuming adequate vitamins and minerals. In some cases, you may be *giving* adequate amounts, but your horse may not be *absorbing* adequate amounts. A hair mineral analysis is a good tool to find out what your horse is absorbing.

If you feel the horse's vitamins and mineral amount is correct and absorption good, but the accessory carpal bone is still not moving easily in all directions, call your certified chiropractor.

▶ When the Checkup is fine, yet symptoms remain, check for:

- Subluxations at: knee, elbow, shoulder (pp. 81, 77, 69)
- Arthritis
- Hoof-wall imbalance

BODY CHECKUP 12
THE SPLINT BONES

I have a theory that the cause of a "popped splint" (the common term for a swelling along the splint bone) may have a chiropractic component. The traditional causes include: trauma, interfering, overwork, unbalanced nutrition, and poor conformation. However, the splint bones can also be subluxated—at least partially. My question is, if the splint bone is aligned properly with its normal flexibility, is it then able to compensate for the extra stress of overuse instead of "popping"?

Almost all of the splint bones I've seen with a popped splint have been subluxated. Certainly the subluxation could have occurred after, or because of, the popped splint. So we have a classic chicken-or-egg

SPLINT BONE CHALLENGE LEVEL ☆☆
Locating Anatomic Area: ☆☆
Positioning of Person or Horse: ☆
Subtle Range of Motion: ☆☆☆
Complex Evaluation of Checkup: ☆☆

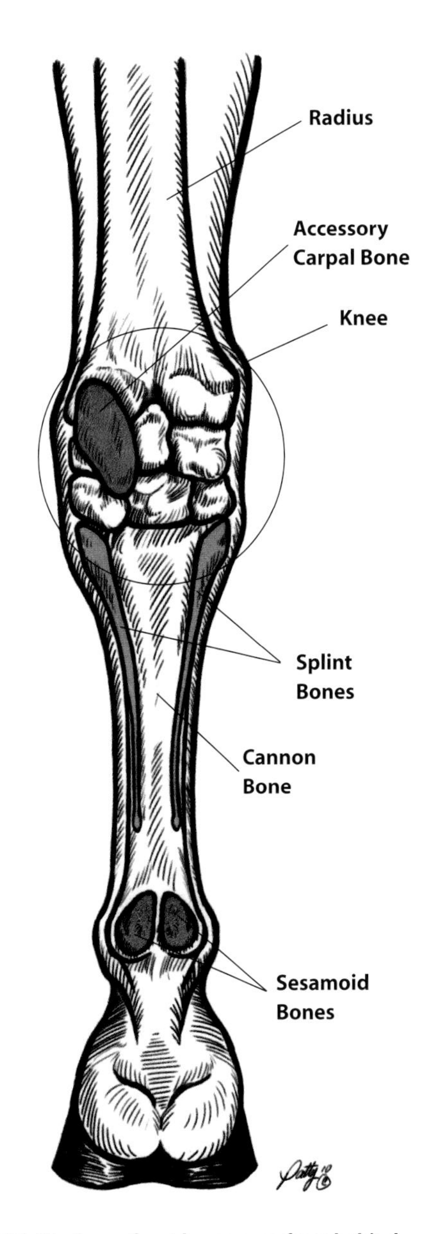

12.1 The lower front leg as seen from behind.

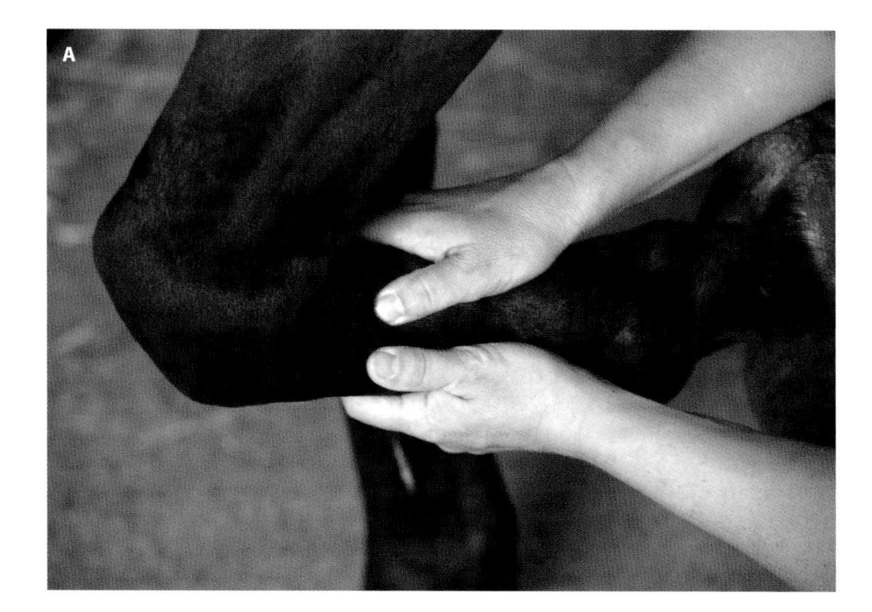

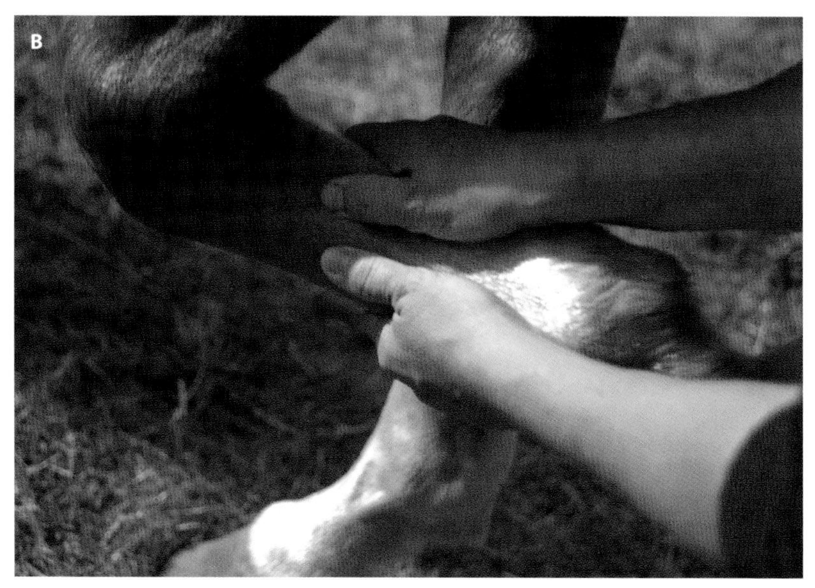

12.2 A & B These two photos of different horses show the position of the hands on the left splint bone of the left front leg for this Checkup. The splint bone is difficult to photograph because it is between the cannon bone and the suspensory ligament.

scenario, with no real way to test it. I am quite confident though, that when you consistently check your horse's splint bones in the way I'm about to explain, you can keep ahead of the game.

Common Symptoms

BEHAVIORAL OR PERFORMANCE SYMPTOMS

Very Common

- Off or short-striding—on a circle only

Frequent

- Short-striding on tight turns

Occasional

- Difficulty with front end lateral work
- Consistent interfering of front legs
- Tripping frequently, usually only on turns

PHYSICAL SYMPTOMS: CURRENT OR PRIOR

- Splint injury, history of
- Strained flexor tendons, history of
- Foot has medial-lateral hoof wall imbalance

Checkup Directions

FUNCTION: There are two splint bones (medial and lateral) on each leg. The function of the splint bones involves the transmission of vertical and rotational forces along the cannon bone. Also, while not an actual "joint," the junction between the splint bones and the cannon bone should be flexible and not "stuck."

RANGE OF MOTION: A splint bone lies on both sides of the cannon bone and is attached to the cannon bone by the interosseous ligament. When there is no calcification in this ligament, the splint bone will gently flex away from the cannon bone in all directions—front, back, up, down, and even in toward the cannon bone. This movement is very small, approximately one-eighth of an inch.

HOW TO

Holding the leg up in a relaxed position, feel just behind the cannon bone and find the splint bone. Place your thumbs on each side of the splint bone (figs. 12.2 A & B). Apply gentle pressure in a side-to-side manner, and you'll feel a small movement as the interosseous ligament gives to the pressure. This is a very subtle movement, approximately one-eighth of an inch. You are feeling for the ability of the splint bone to "give" to this pressure, rather than a sensation of pushing on a solid, immoveable rock.

Apply side-to-side pressure all along the splint bone from top to bottom. It's normal for the bottom one-third to be "looser" than the top two-thirds. The bottom part of the splint bone may move as much as one-quarter inch.

Also check for the same subtle "give" as you push the entire splint bone up toward the knee and down toward the fetlock. This same give should also be felt as you push the splint bone directly in toward the cannon bone.

Be sure to check both medial and lateral (right and left) splint bones on all legs.

Diagnosis

When you do not feel the subtle one-eighth give from side to side of the splint bone, it is likely subluxated. If you do not feel the gentle give in all directions (and there is no history of a popped splint—see below), the splint bone is subluxated.

It is important to note that if there has been a previous popped splint, there may be no movement in that segment of the splint bone, as the interosseous ligament often calcifies in a traumatically injured area. There may, in fact, be no movement in the entire splint bone, depending on the severity of the injury.

Summary: SPLINT BONE

- When a splint bone is subluxated, there are often other subluxations, so check the knee, accessory carpal bone, and fetlock (pp. 81, 84, 90) before calling chiropractor.
- When the Checkup is fine, but symptoms remain, check for:
    - Subluxations at: knee, accessory carpal bone, fetlock, shoulder, shoulder blade, ribs under the shoulder (pp. 81, 84, 90, 69, 66, 117)
    - Vitamin or mineral imbalance
    - Hoof-wall imbalance
    - Heel-pain syndrome

BODY CHECKUP 13
THE FETLOCK

I did a quick Body Checkup on a five-year-old Thoroughbred hunter mare that was on a two-week trial period prior to purchase. I found some lumbar subluxations, but what concerned me more was the amount of back-muscle tightness I noted in her: It was much more than I would have expected from the subluxations.

As I finished checking the mare's legs, I was quite surprised to find both her front fetlocks had at least 50 percent less range of motion than normal. They should have easily bent up toward her knees when I picked up her front feet. They didn't! They only bent about halfway before they felt "frozen" in place. I believe that her back muscles had become so tight due to her need to compensate for her fetlock problem.

The potential owner was happy I discovered this problem, saving her close to $1,000 in veterinary pre-purchase exams and X-rays. There was no way this mare could have held up to a rigorous jumping schedule without normal fetlock flexion. The mare went on to find a happy home where there was no jumping involved.

FETLOCK CHALLENGE LEVEL ☆
Locating Anatomic Area: ☆
Positioning of Person or Horse: ☆
Subtle Range of Motion: ☆
Complex Evaluation of Checkup: ☆

Common Symptoms

BEHAVIOR OR PERFORMANCE SYMPTOMS

Very Common

- Decreased flexion of fetlock
- Tripping in front
- Feet landing toe first
- Reluctance to jump
- Stumbling on tight turns or around barrels

Frequent

- Stiff in the front end
- Difficulty with turns

Occasional

- Struggles with front end lateral work
- Short-striding, or "off" in front

PHYSICAL SYMPTOMS: CURRENT OR PRIOR

- Ligament strain, history of
- Heels, tendency to grow to excess

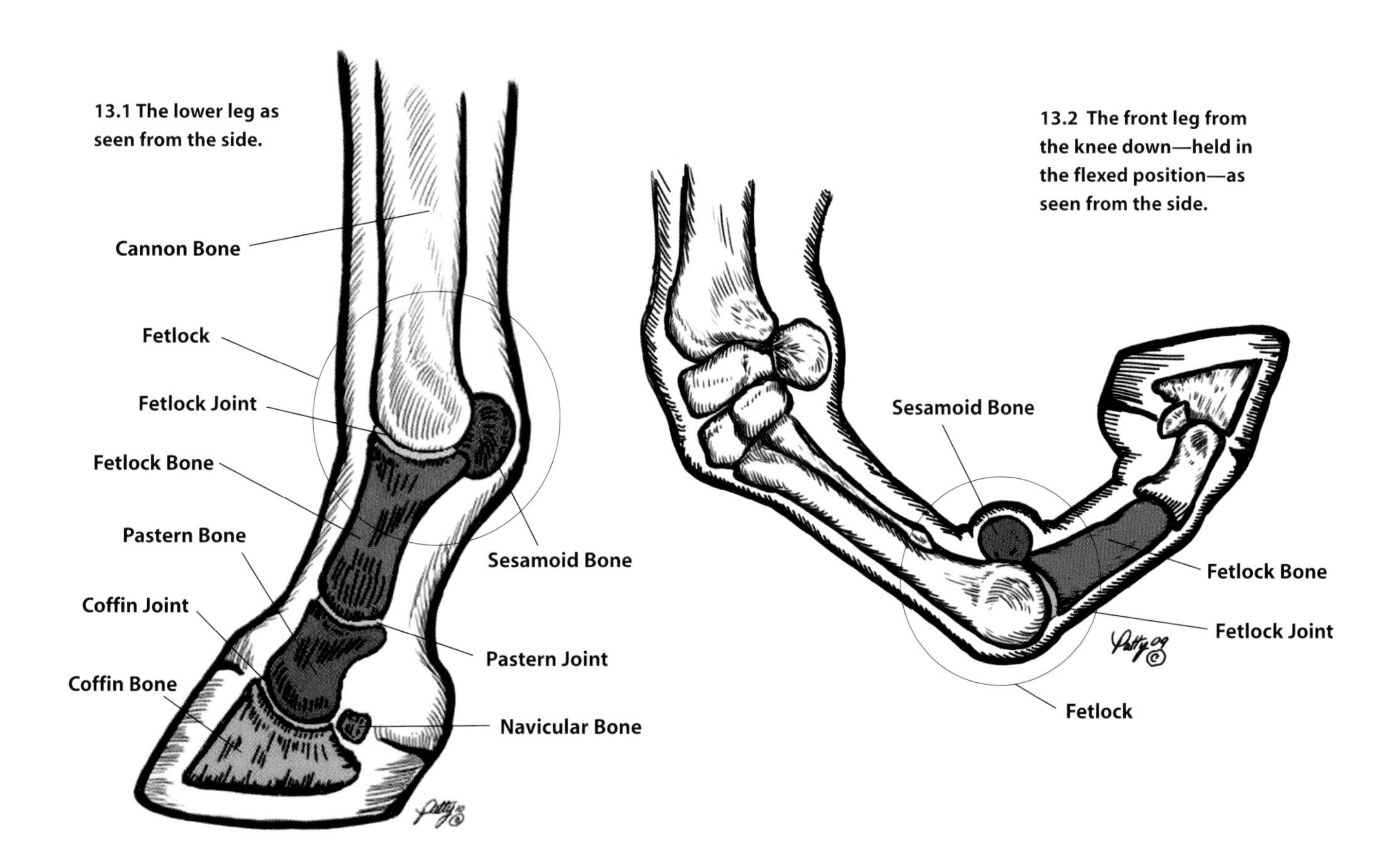

13.1 The lower leg as seen from the side.

13.2 The front leg from the knee down—held in the flexed position—as seen from the side.

Checkup Directions

FUNCTION: The fetlock facilitates force coming from the ground and traveling up the leg properly (acts as a shock absorber) and also helps with flexion in the front leg.

RANGE OF MOTION: The fetlock's normal range is quite large. When the horse is standing with his legs perpendicular to the ground, the fetlock is forward approximately 45 degrees. When flexed, the fetlock angle should move approximately 75 degrees to the back.

HOW TO

First, pick up one of the horse's legs, and be sure the entire leg is relaxed (fig. 13.3). Sometimes a horse, expecting you to clean out his foot, tries to be "helpful" by holding up his leg up for you, so wait a minute or so until he relaxes his whole leg and lets you hold it up. Then check the fetlock range of motion by holding the toe of the hoof and watching how far it automatically flexes, followed by adding pressure until it stops flexing while supporting the horse's leg with your free hand (figs. 13.4 A & B).

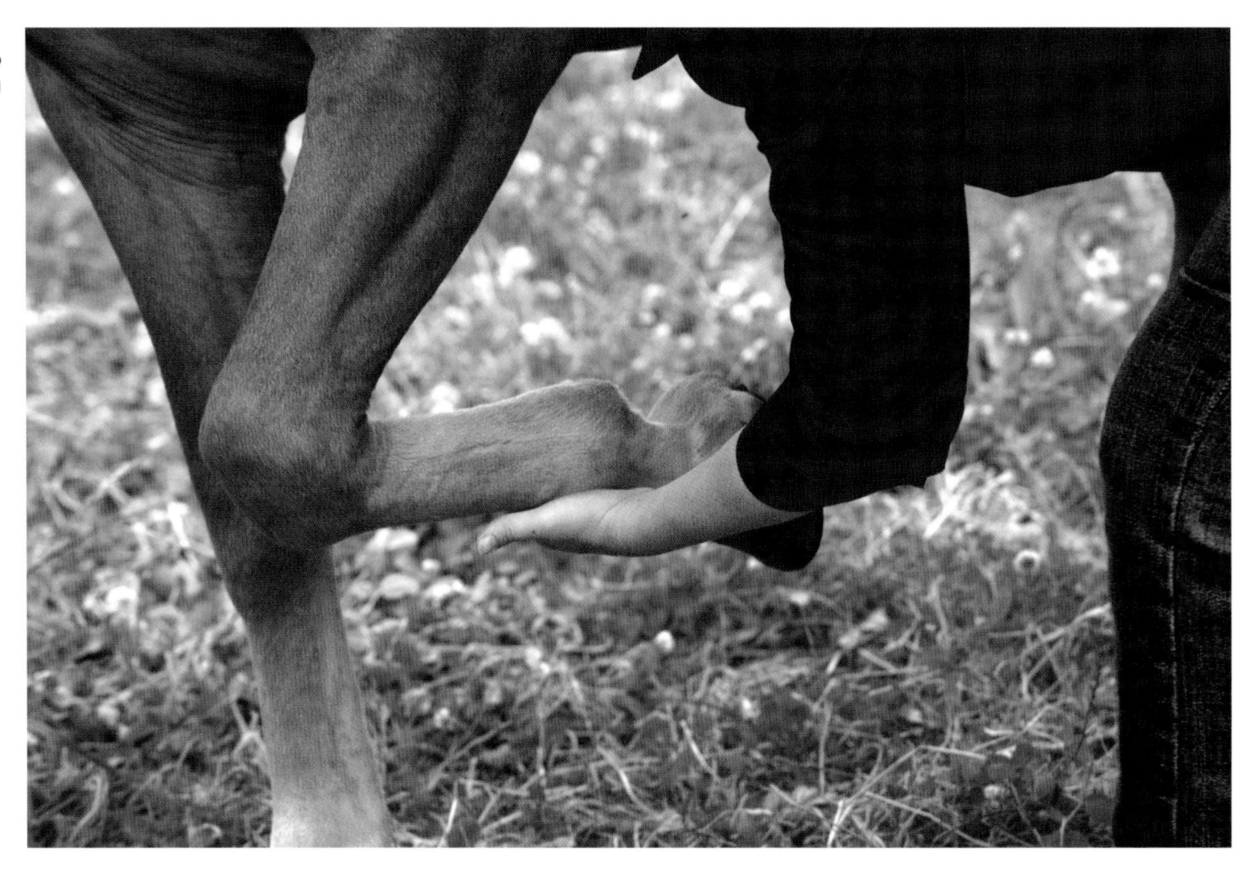

13.3 Allow the horse to relax his leg into your hand.

Diagnosis

When the fetlock does not flex comfortably through the entire range of motion, it may need adjusting. Or, it may have a decreased range of motion because of arthritis, tendon stiffness or adhesions, or sesamoid bone subluxations.

Compare both front fetlocks. If they have the same amount of flexion, you typically do not have a chiropractic issue. Check the fetlocks in the hind legs, as well.

Summary: FETLOCK

- When subluxation diagnosed (uncommon), call chiropractor.
- Checkup is fine, but symptoms remain, check for:
  - Subluxation: sesamoid bones (p. 94)
  - Fetlock arthritis
  - Hoof-wall imbalance
  - Mineral or vitamin imbalance
  - Early flexor tendon strain
  - Heel-pain syndrome
  - "Joint mice" in fetlock

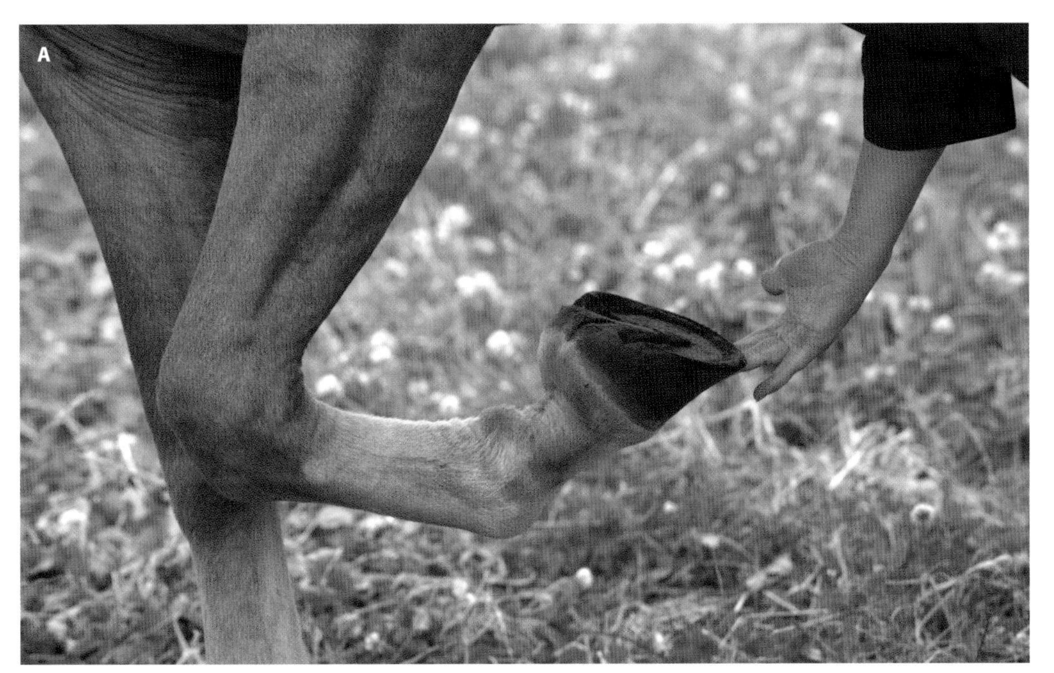

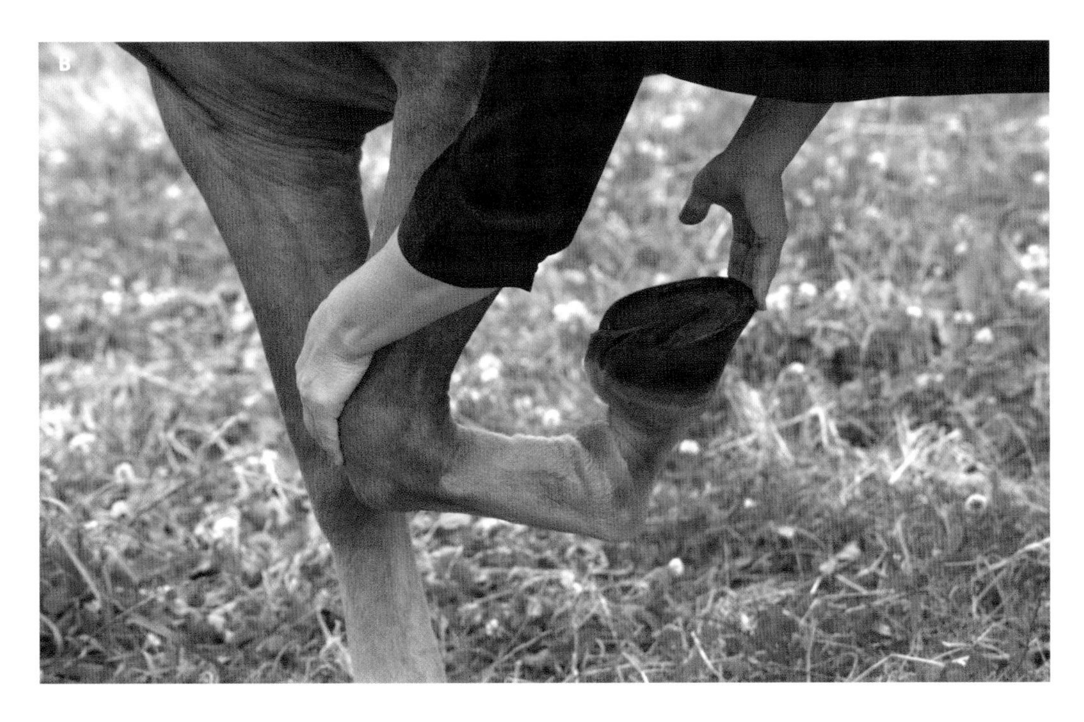

13.4 A & B
This horse has perfect fetlock flexion. In A, the fetlock automatically flexes simply by holding the leg up by the toe of the hoof, while B shows the fetlock fully flexed.

BODY CHECKUP 14 THE SESAMOID BONES

One of my clients asked me to check her three-year-old Paint filly, Teacup. She was a very cute and flashy Western Pleasure horse. Her owner, Jamie, noticed that when trotting to the left on a circle, she would become slightly lame. This was a subtle lameness, one that the average horseperson could miss. But Jamie had lots of experience and always tried to catch things early before they got worse.

Typically, any "offness" that is more noticeable at a trot rather than a walk is a "leg issue," and I usually suggest clients start with their traditional veterinarian in such cases. However, in Teacup's case, I knew that this leg problem was so subtle it would be difficult for traditional diagnostics to solve.

Upon examining Teacup, I only found a single chiropractic subluxation: her left lateral (left) sesamoid bone. "Well, Jamie," I said, "that's all I can find. Let's see if she's changed at all now that she's been adjusted."

We put her back on the left circle and the offness was gone. It was rather surprising. On checking the shape of her foot, I found that the side-to-side hoof-wall balance was incorrect, which was throwing her sesamoid bone out of adjustment. We regularly adjusted her sesamoid as her hoof-wall balance was corrected over a few trims, and she did fine.

It is rewarding to see how fixing one little subluxation can sometimes make such a big difference!

SESAMOID BONE CHALLENGE LEVEL ☆☆☆
Locating Anatomic Area: ☆
Positioning of Person or Horse: ☆
Subtle Range of Motion: ☆☆☆
Complex Evaluation of Checkup: ☆☆

Common Symptoms

BEHAVIORAL OR PERFORMANCE SYMPTOMS

Very Common

- Difficulty with fetlock flexion

Frequent

- Short-striding or "off" in front, possibly only on a circle

Occasional

- Reluctance to jump
- Going wide on barrel turns
- Difficulty with tight turns
- Difficulty with lateral movements
- Feet landing toe first
- Tripping

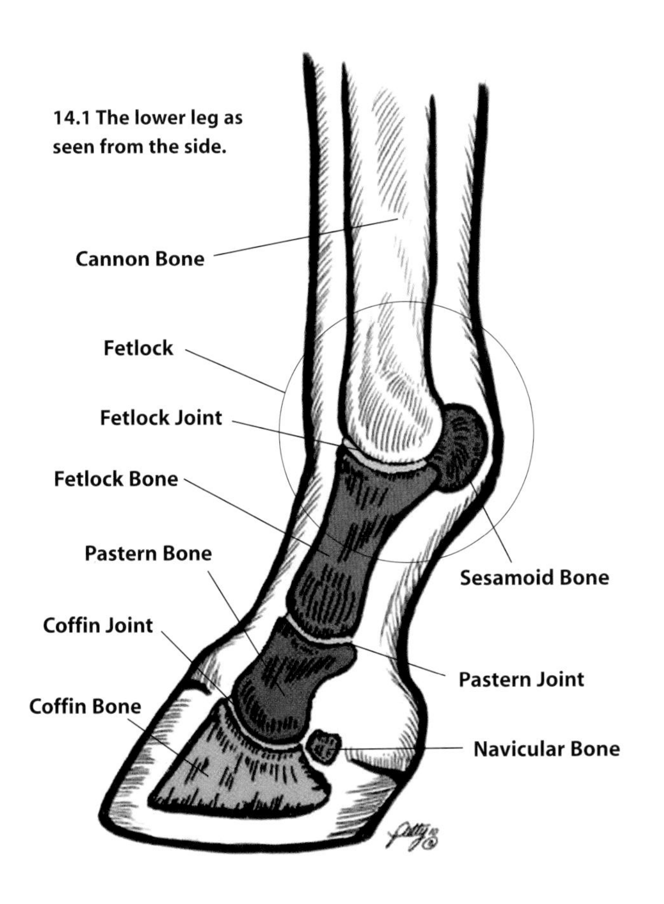

14.1 The lower leg as seen from the side.

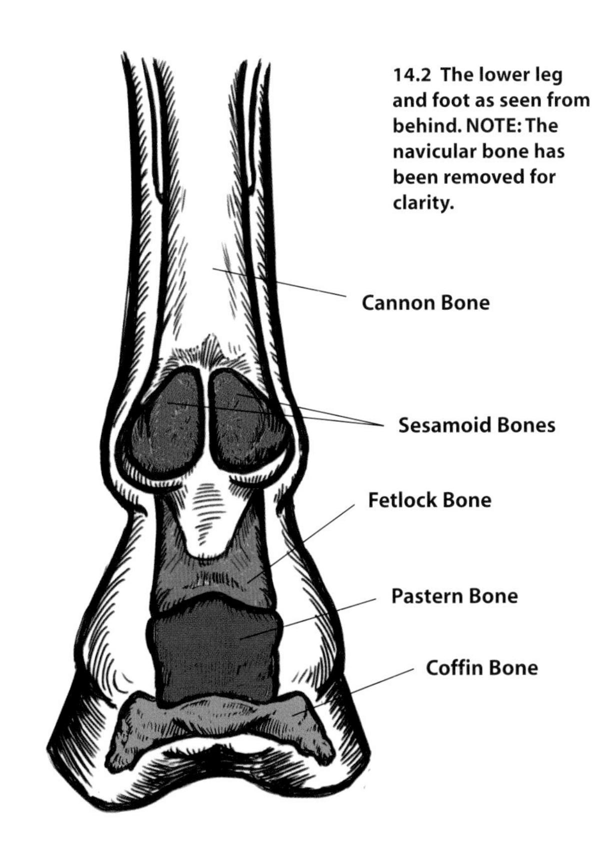

14.2 The lower leg and foot as seen from behind. NOTE: The navicular bone has been removed for clarity.

PHYSICAL SYMPTOMS: CURRENT OR PRIOR

- Medial-to-lateral (left-to-right) hoof-wall imbalance, history of
- Foot is "clubby" or has tendency to grow excess heel

Checkup Directions

FUNCTION: The sesamoid bones function as part of the shock-absorbing mechanism of the front legs and are also a weight and power transition point.

RANGE OF MOTION: Because the sesamoid bones help transmit weight and power from the cannon bone to the fetlock and navicular bones, in all directions, they need to be mobile in all directions. Their normal range of motion is most simply described as a circle. A sesamoid bone can move approximately one-eighth to one-quarter inch in each direction from its normal position.

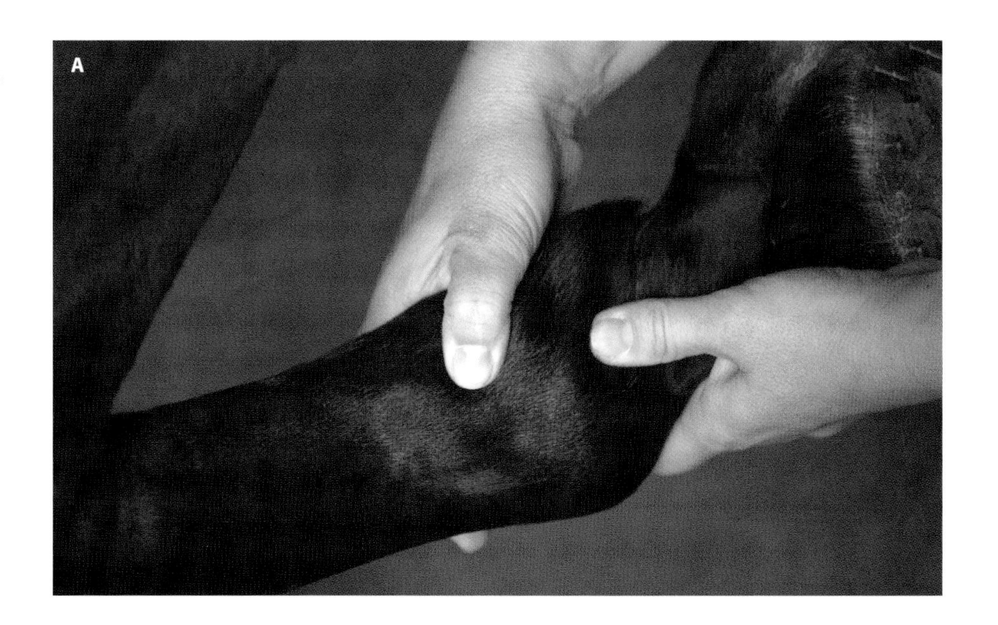

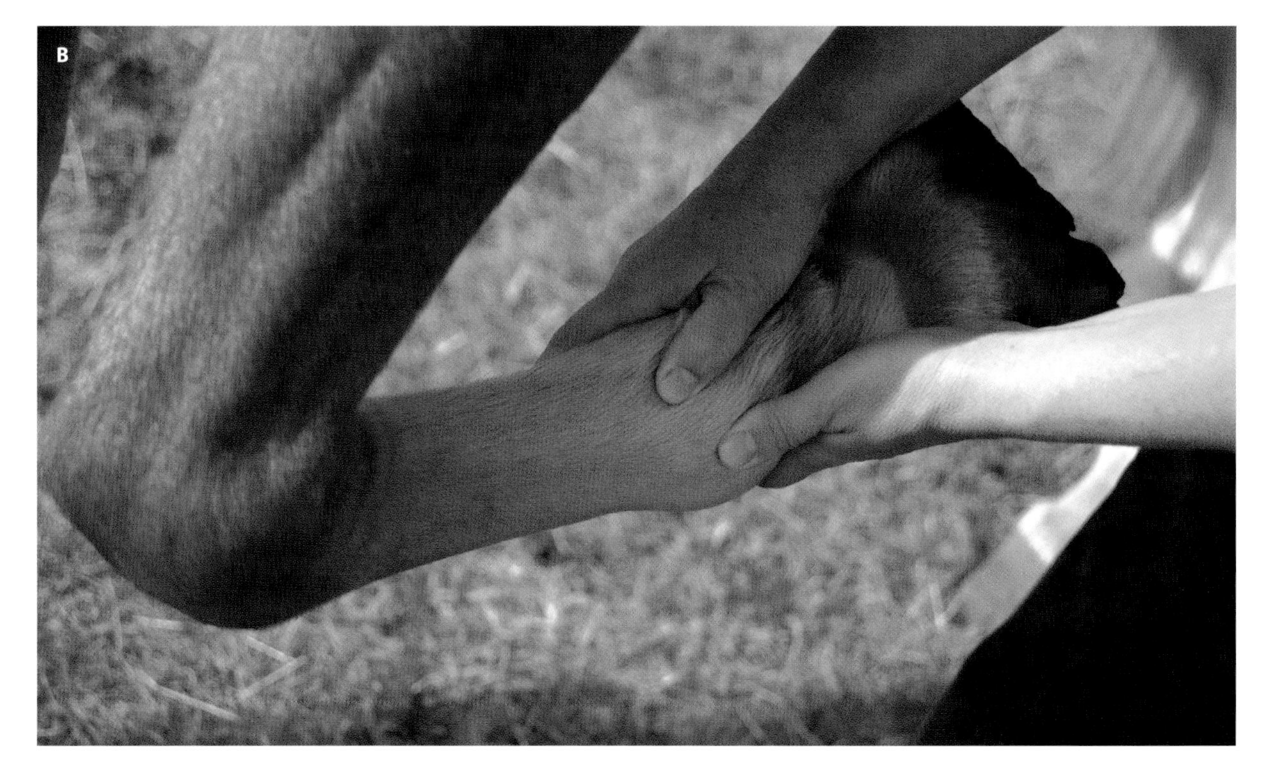

14.3 A & B These two photos show different views of me examining two different horses' sesamoid bones, located on the back of the fetlock. The sesamoid bones are most easily felt with the leg held up off the ground as shown here.

HOW TO

Hold one of the horse's feet up with the leg completely relaxed from the shoulder down. Cup the fetlock with both hands so that your thumbs rest on each side of the sesamoid bone being examined (figs. 14.3 A & B).

Gently slide the sesamoid bone in a circular manner as if you were sliding it around the face of a clock. Do not use additional force if you encounter resistance in any area. The movement is very subtle. As mentioned, the normal range is from one-eighth to one-quarter inch. The key is in the smoothness of this movement. The sesamoid should slide easily along its path, rather than "sticking" or being more difficult to move in any section.

Diagnosis

When there is any "stickiness" in the movement and the bone does not glide easily in all directions, it is most often a chiropractic subluxation. Be sure to check both right and left (medial and lateral) sesamoid bones on both front and rear legs. Compare the front legs and rear legs separately since front and rear sesamoid bones have different ranges of motion.

Summary: SESAMOID BONES

- When subluxation apparent, check the fetlock, pastern, coffin joint, and knee (pp. 90, 98, 102, 81) since sesamoid bones rarely subluxate on their own, then call chiropractor.
- When no movement in a sesamoid bone, call veterinarian to X-ray for old fractures and/or calcification of ligaments.
- When Checkup is clear, yet symptoms remain, check for:
  - Hoof-wall imbalance
  - Mineral or vitamin deficiency
  - Arthritis in fetlock, knee, or coffin bone
  - Early tendon strain

BODY CHECKUP 15
THE PASTERN

I've worked on only a handful of Akhal-Tekes. They've all been interesting, to say the least. I examined one mare that was very short-strided when compared to what was expected given her breeding and build.

Her name was Matilda and she was about eight years old. With a different owner, she had been used as a reiner but was now working as an eventer.

I had adjusted Matilda a few times in the past. Each time her fluidity and stride length would improve, but it would slowly erode over the weeks that followed. In addition, her feet "angles" were not satisfactory to her owner, despite the farrier doing his best. She never seemed perfectly comfortable "in her feet," and the angle of her shoulder was extremely straight. Yet, after I adjusted her, she didn't move like a horse with these issues, she strode out well and appeared comfortable.

One day I got a chance to chat with the farrier. He explained some of the difficulty with her feet. "It's like she grows more heel than toe, and—ever so slightly—puts her toe down first when she walks," he said.

"That makes sense to me," I replied, "because that's how her pastern movement feels. Ever so slightly, not quite right. But both feet are the same, so I concluded that the 'not quite right' feeling was due to her very upright pasterns."

At that point we recommended to the owner that the veterinarian be called out to evaluate and possibly X-ray the pasterns. Sadly, it turned out that there were bone chips ("joint mice") from her pastern bones affecting the coffin joints. Joint mice often don't cause problems, but in Matilda's case, they resulted in changes in her foot and leg joint angles.

Once this was diagnosed, Matilda was kept on joint supplements, trimmed every six weeks like clockwork, and given chiropractic care to keep her front end as "lined up" as possible. With this maintenance schedule, she continued to perform very well.

PASTERN CHALLENGE LEVEL ☆☆☆
Locating Anatomic Area: ☆
Positioning of Person or Horse: ☆
Subtle Range of Motion: ☆☆☆
Complex Evaluation of Checkup: ☆

Common Symptoms

BEHAVIORAL OR PERFORMANCE SYMPTOMS

Very Common

- Stumbling with front feet

Frequent

- Feet landing toe first
- Decreased fetlock flexion

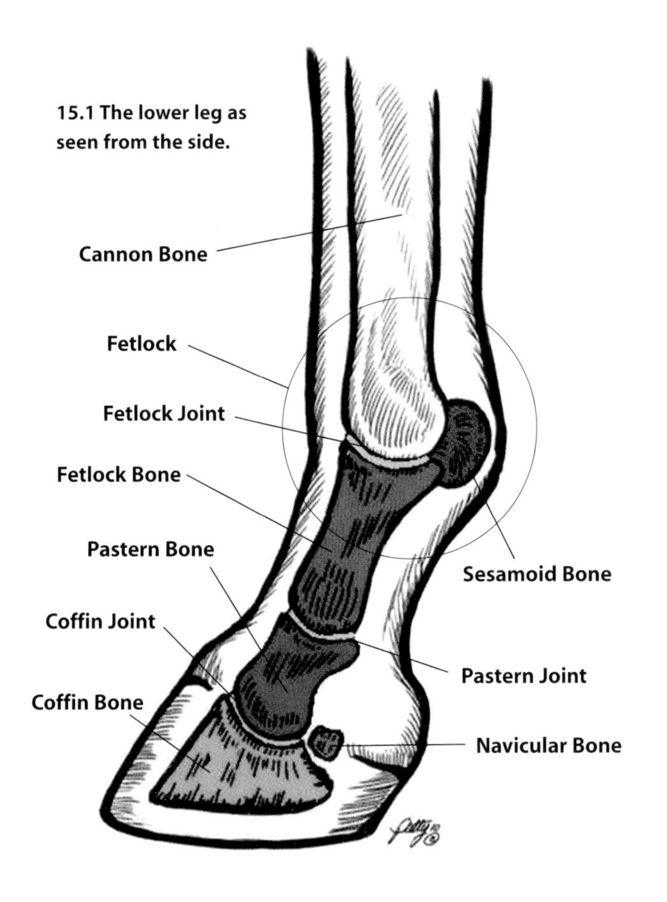

15.1 The lower leg as seen from the side.

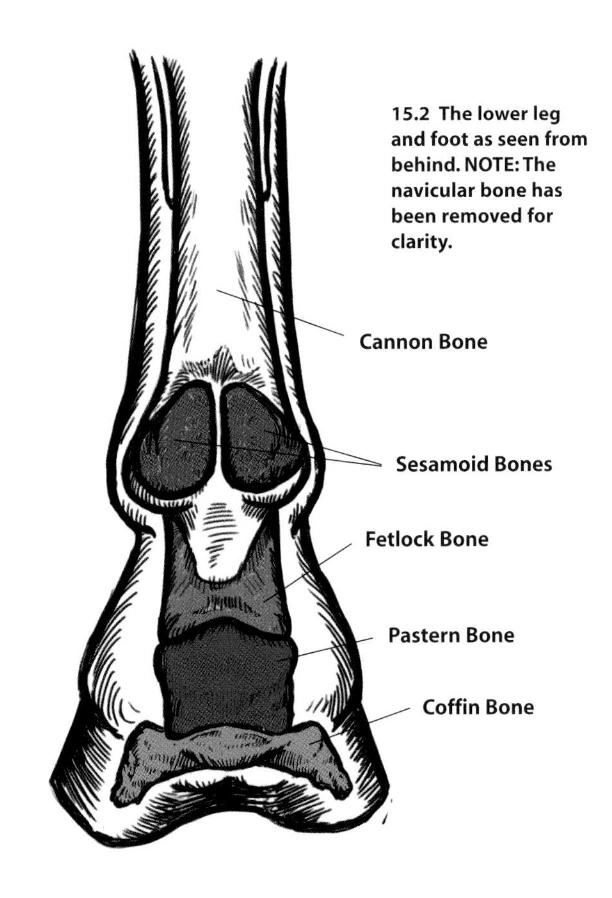

15.2 The lower leg and foot as seen from behind. NOTE: The navicular bone has been removed for clarity.

Occasional

- Difficulty with tight turns
- Unwillingness to jump
- Short-striding—front end
- Front-end stiffness
- Tripping

PHYSICAL SYMPTOMS: CURRENT OR PRIOR

- "Tender-footed," especially with no apparent conformational cause
- Foot has medial-to-lateral hoof-wall imbalance
- Front feet have "high-heel/ low-heel" syndrome

Checkup Directions

FUNCTION: The pastern helps with transference of the concussive forces from the ground, from the coffin bone to fetlock bone. It also helps with lower-limb flexion.

RANGE OF MOTION: The pastern joint best shows chiropractic abnormalities when you check its ability to twist to each side. The normal "twisting" ability of the pastern joint is approximately one-half inch maximum to each side.

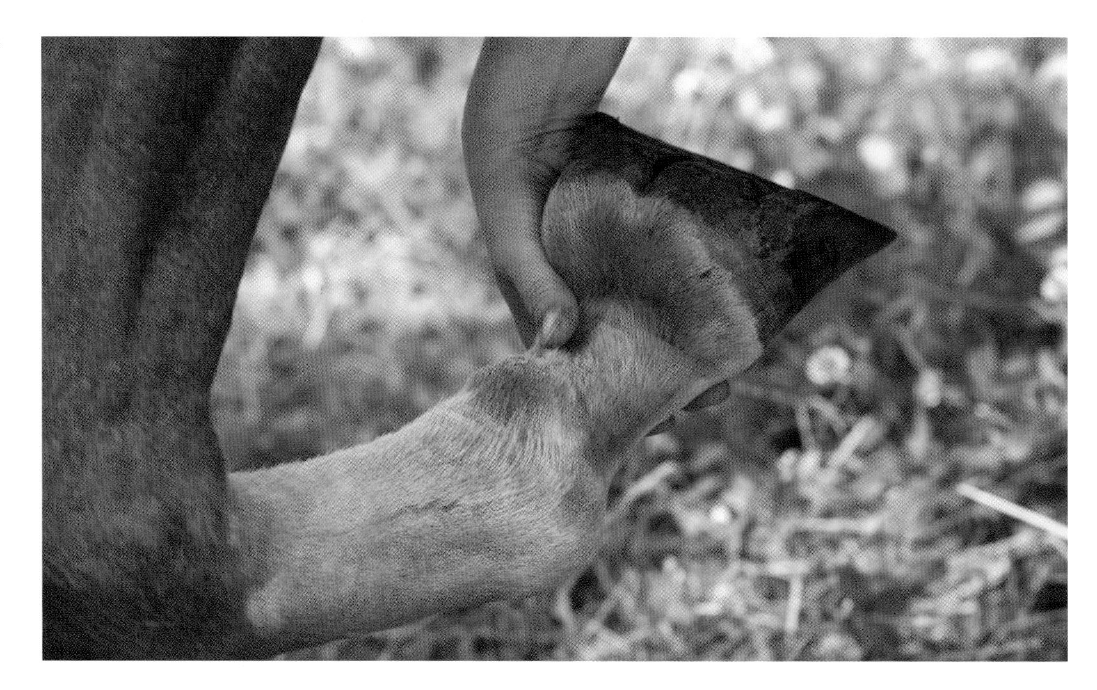

15.3 The placement of the lower hand for this Body Checkup.

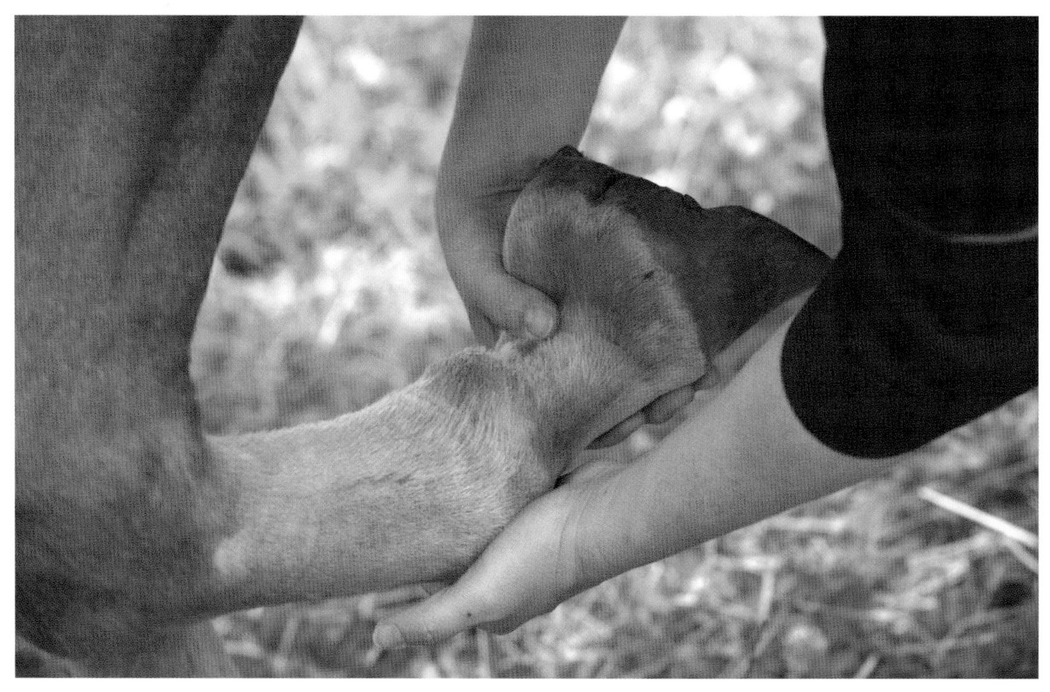

15.4 The placement of the upper hand for this Body Checkup.

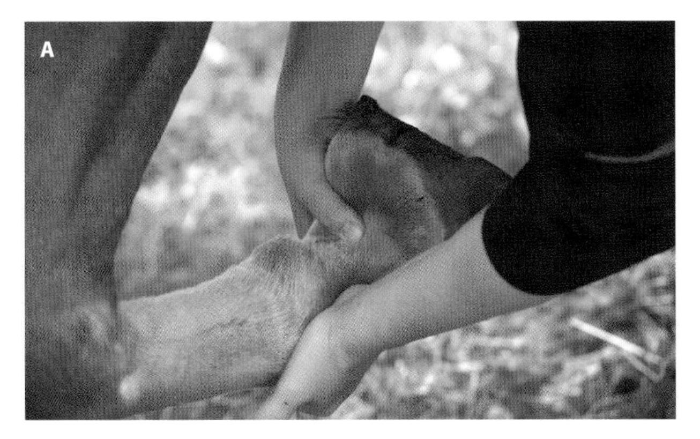

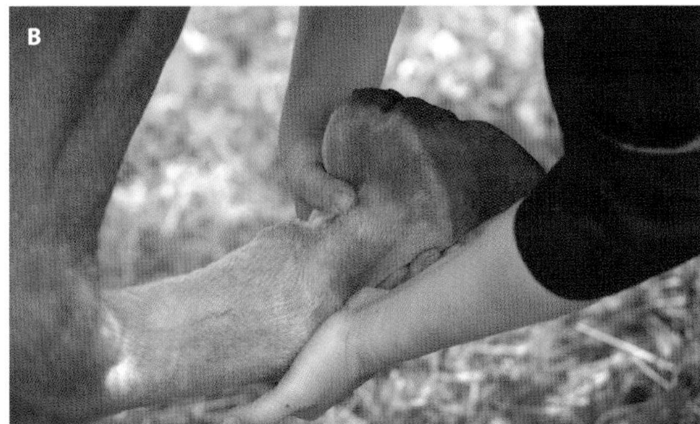

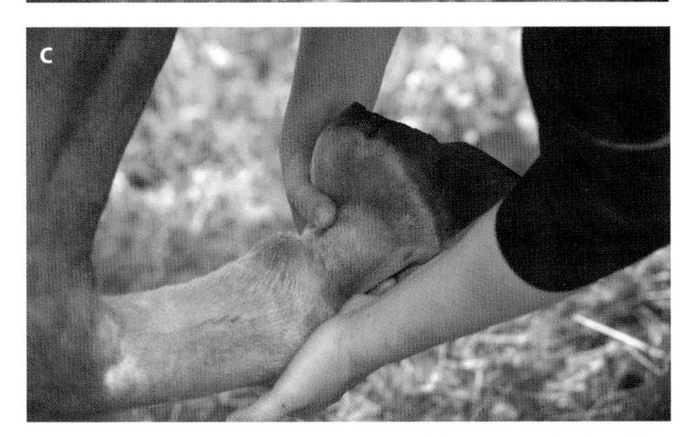

15.5 A–C I demonstrate the movement of the pastern during this Body Checkup. Although the movement is small and not obvious in the photos, you can see the change in position of my thumb. It moves from an inward position in A, to a neutral position in B, and an outward position in C. My hand did not move on the hoof, but rather the pastern joint was "twisted" to each side.

HOW TO

While holding the leg up in a relaxed position, place one hand on the pastern bone. Because of its small size, I recommend holding it with your first two fingers and thumb, while letting the rest of your hand rest on the hoof wall (fig. 15.3). With your other hand, hold onto the fetlock joint and keep it from moving (fig. 15.4).

Next, gently twist the pastern bone from one side to the other. You want to observe a nice, flexible twist that is the same going to both sides (figs. 15.5 A–C).

Diagnosis

When the pastern does not twist symmetrically to each side, you may have a chiropractic subluxation.

Summary: PASTERN

- When you suspect a subluxation, check fetlock, sesamoid bones, and coffin joint (pp. 90, 94, 102) since pasterns rarely subluxate on their own, then call chiropractor.
- When the Checkup is clear, yet symptoms remain, check for:
  - Heel-pain syndrome
  - Hoof-wall imbalance
  - Early tendon strain
  - Laminitis/founder, history of
  - "Joint mice" in pastern joint
  - Arthritis

BODY CHECKUP 16 THE COFFIN JOINT

Living with a horse that has gone through an episode of founder (laminitis), can be challenging. It takes a special person to maintain the care needed to keep these horses from foundering all over again.

I met one such owner, Megan, and her horse Blue, a palomino with blue eyes. He was a 17-hand, heavy, big boned, Quarter Horse. Did I mention he was big? In fact, he was so overweight—with enough fat to create a 1½-inch-deep trough down his back—that I was shocked to find out that he was not foundering right then. He had foundered about two years earlier, and Megan had nursed him back to health. Apparently, Blue was now "much thinner" and able to walk about comfortably, although he wouldn't move faster than a walk.

Megan called me out as part of her concern for his overall health: During his bout with laminitis, he had lain on the ground for months. X-rays of his feet were fine, but she wanted to make sure that his body was in alignment after all that stress and pain. She thought general body discomfort might be the reason why Blue refused to go faster than the walk.

Blue had a lot of subluxations along his thoracic spine, and also his ribs. These adjusted quite readily. Interestingly enough, his coffin joints were fine and quite mobile; I would have expected some kind of change in them with the history of founder. After his adjustment, Blue walked with much more fluidity: His very large rear end swayed side to side instead of being completely stiff. But he still didn't want to go faster than a walk.

So we did a series of acupuncture treatments for his feet. Afterward, Blue began to trot, even uphill and downhill! It is my hope that Megan will be able to ride Blue soon to help get him back in healthy shape.

COFFIN JOINT CHALLENGE LEVEL ☆☆☆☆
Locating Anatomic Area: ☆
Positioning of Horse or Handler: ☆
Subtle Range of Motion: ☆☆☆☆
Complex Evaluation of Checkup: ☆☆☆☆

Common Symptoms

BEHAVIORAL OR PERFORMANCE SYMPTOMS

Very Common

- Stiff in front
- Unwillingness to jump

Frequent

- Short-striding in front
- Difficulty with turns
- Feet landing toe first

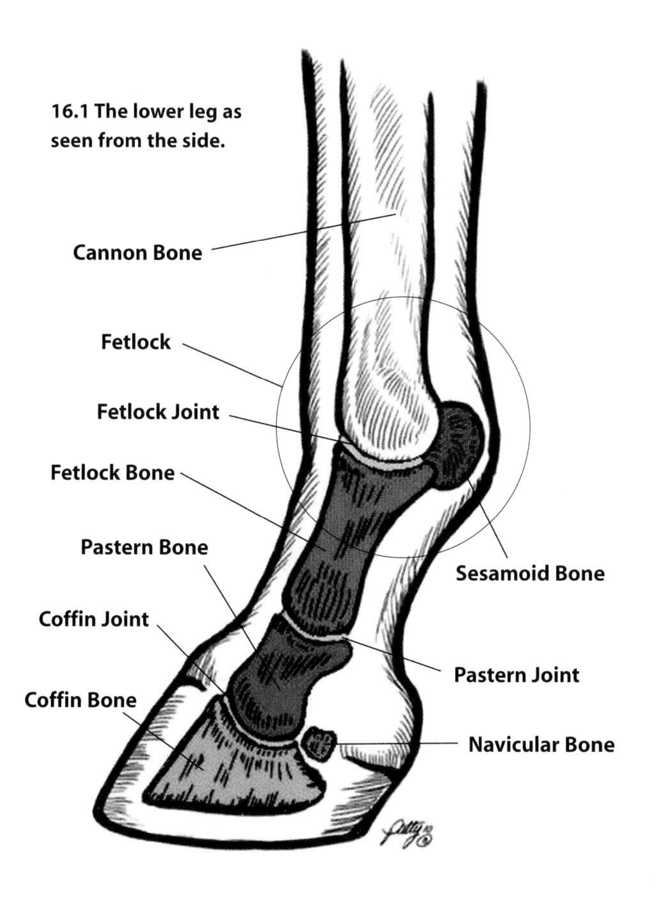

16.1 The lower leg as seen from the side.

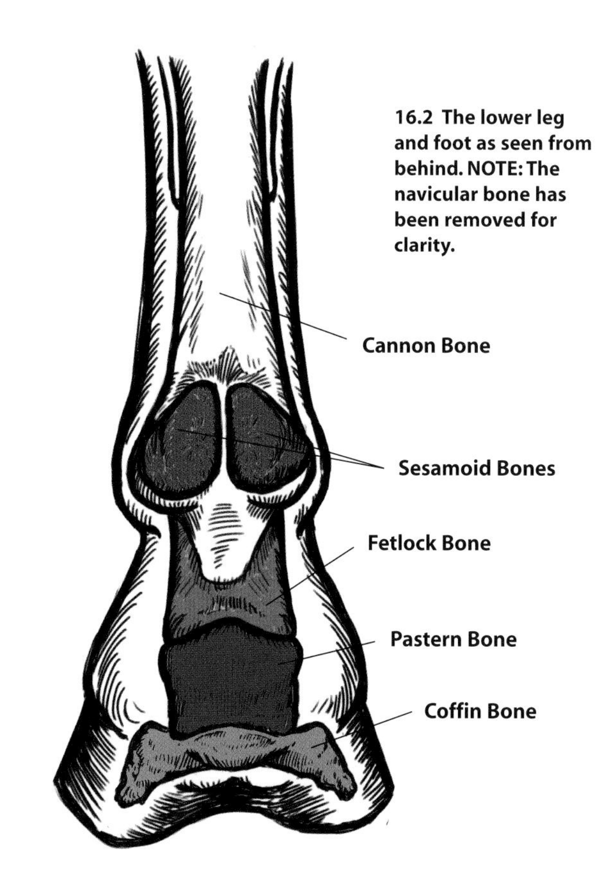

16.2 The lower leg and foot as seen from behind. NOTE: The navicular bone has been removed for clarity.

Occasional

- Unwillingness to go downhill
- Tripping

PHYSICAL SYMPTOMS: CURRENT OR PRIOR

- Laminitis
- High-heel/low-heel syndrome
- "Tender-footed," especially with no apparent conformational cause
- Medial-to-lateral hoof-wall imbalance

Checkup Directions

FUNCTION: The coffin bone is the first bone to receive the ground forces of the hoof and it transmits those forces up the leg. The attachment of the coffin bone to the hoof wall is a complex mechanism of internal hoof structures involving cartilage and laminae. The cartilage and laminae enable the hoof to twist side to side.

RANGE OF MOTION: Because you are checking a joint that is inside the hoof capsule, this Checkup is an approximation of the coffin joint's true range of

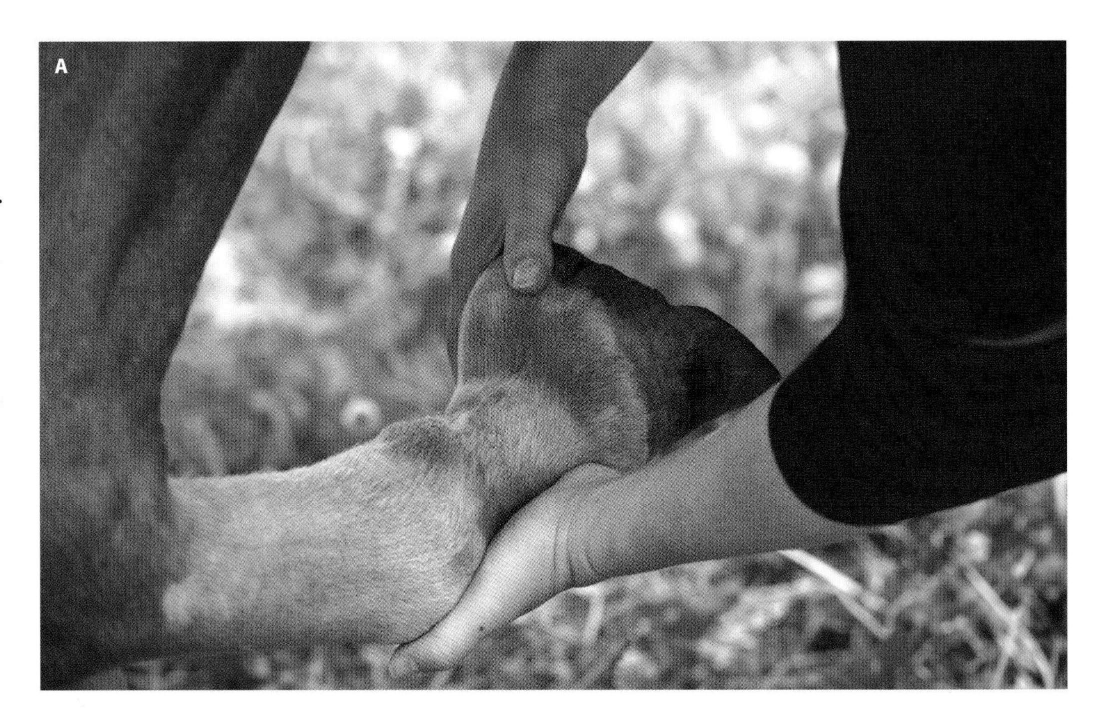

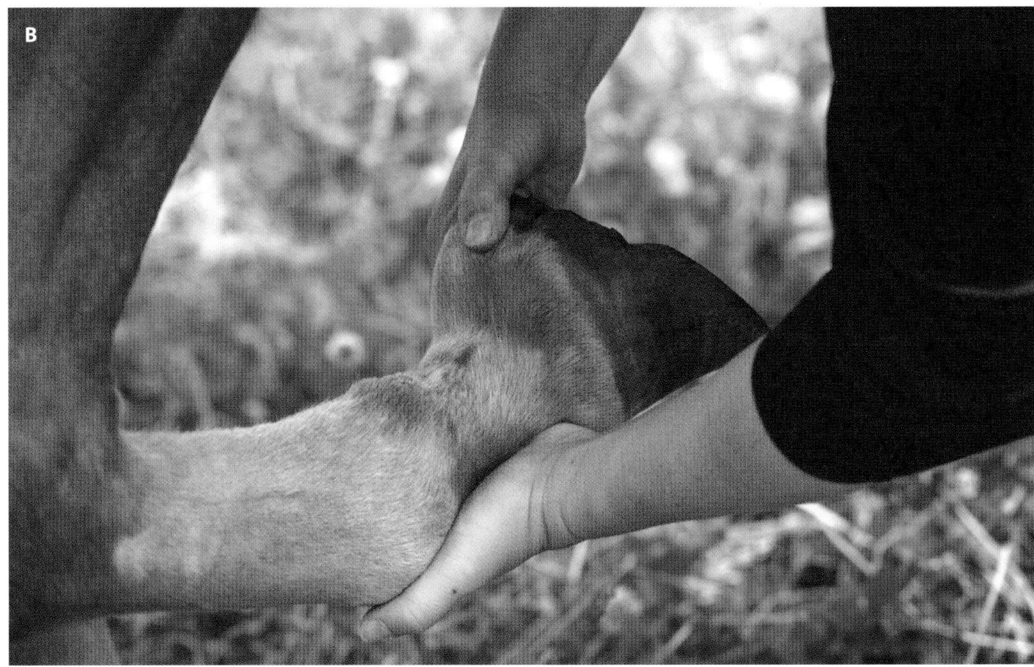

16.3 A & B **The movement of the coffin joint is not obvious in these photos, but notice the change in position of my thumb. In A, the thumb appears more inward, showing the coffin-joint movement to the left. In B, it appears more outward, showing the coffin-joint movement to the right.**

motion. Average normal range of motion is anywhere from one-half to 1 1/2 inches of hoof movement.

HOW TO

With the horse's leg held up in a relaxed position, place one hand just above the coffin joint on the front of the leg. With your other hand, gently twist the hoof to one side and then the other (figs. 16.3 A & B).

As you come to the end of the coffin joint's range of motion, there is a soft "end-feel," which is simply how the joint feels at the end of its range of motion. It is possible to twist the hoof further after the end-feel, but at that point you are feeling the additional range of motion of the internal hoof structures, not just the coffin joint. Be sure you only evaluate the range of motion of the coffin joint up to the first, soft, end-feel. NOTE: Sometimes when the internal hoof structures (most notably the lateral cartilages) have calcified (usually with age), there will not be a soft "end-feel."

Diagnosis

Usually, where there is more movement of the hoof to one side than the other, there is a coffin bone subluxation. With no or minimal movement to either side, it is typically arthritis.

Summary: COFFIN JOINT

- When you suspect a subluxation: With younger horse with no history of arthritis, call chiropractor; with older horse, check with veterinarian for arthritis or calcification of lateral cartilages.
- When no indication of subluxation but symptoms remain, check for:
    - Hoof-wall imbalance
    - Arthritis
    - Laminitis/founder, subclinical
    - Heel-pain syndrome
    - Early tendon strain

Section 3

THE BACK BODY CHECKUPS

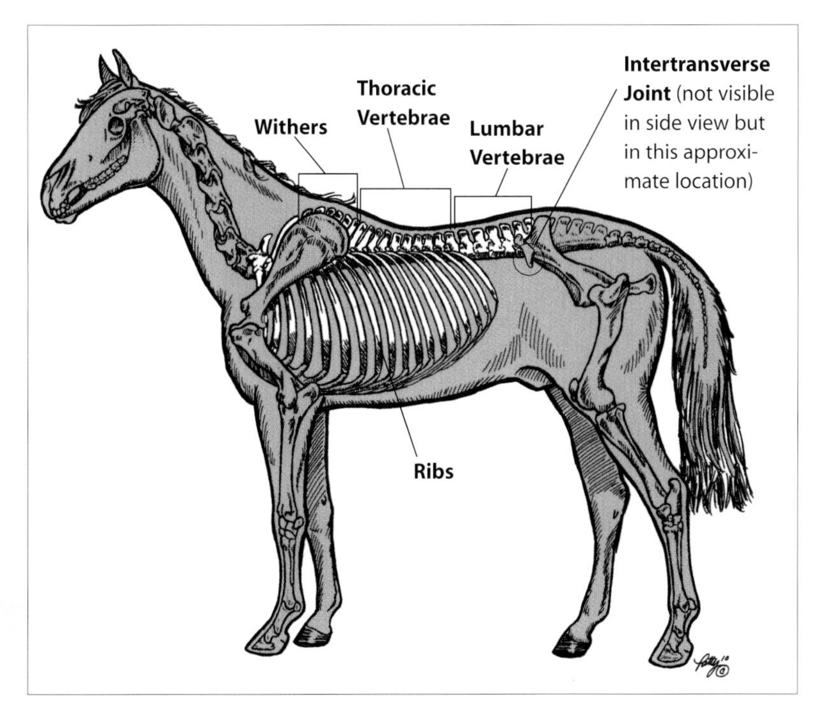

The Back Body Checkup areas.

Back Problems: General Symptoms

- Cold-backed
- Stiff, but may often warm up to perform acceptably
- Difficulty bending in one or both directions
- Short-striding in front or rear
- "Girthy"/"cinchy"
- Difficulty with collection and/or impulsion
- Unable to stand still, especially when being mounted
- Hypersensitivity to brushing
- Rolling excessively
- Crow-hopping or bucking
- Drops shoulder on turns
- Goes wide on turns
- Difficulty using topline muscles properly
- Difficulty holding the hind feet up for farrier
- Consistently resting one hind leg (either the same leg or alternating)
- Difficulty cantering/loping in one or both directions
- Cannot track straight
- Difficulty with gait transitions
- Has trouble picking up, maintaining, or changing leads

BODY CHECKUP 17
THE WITHERS

The withers are often subluxated on the left side, primarily because we mount and dismount from that side. Do you know why we get on and off from the left? It has been said it was because right-handed people had their sword belted on their left side. Obviously, this would have made it difficult to get on from the right.

Unless you are still carrying a sword, please do make a point of getting on and off from both sides of the horse. In addition, use a mounting block—mounting the horse pulls on the withers, and can subluxate them over time. A special note to ropers: Roping horses frequently have chronically sore withers, unfortunately due to the "jerk" inherent in roping work. If you are a roper, it is to your advantage to learn some massage techniques, as well as to have your horse regularly adjusted. Good saddle pads and correct saddle fit also help, but your horse still needs regular bodywork to keep from becoming sore and sour over time.

WITHERS CHALLENGE LEVEL ☆☆
Locating Anatomic Area: ☆
Positioning of Horse or Handler: ☆
Subtle Range of Motion: ☆☆
Complex Evaluation of Checkup: ☆☆

Common Symptoms

BEHAVIORAL OR PERFORMANCE SYMPTOMS

Very Common

- Difficulty with lateral-bending movements in the front end
- Difficulty with collection and impulsion

Frequent

- Stiff front end
- Reluctance to stand still, especially when being mounted

Occasional

- Short-striding in front
- "Girthy"/"cinchy"
- Cold-backed
- Tripping

PHYSICAL SYMPTOMS: CURRENT OR PRIOR

- Shoulder or shoulder-blade range of motion, decreased
- Shoulder blade high on one side
- Shoulders seem tight and difficult to move or stretch
- Muscles tight around shoulder-blade area
- Hypersensitivity to being brushed
- Rider feels crooked or saddle slips to one side
- Trouble with saddle fit

- Ewe neck
- Struggle to develop topline muscles

Checkup Directions

FUNCTION: The withers are the spinous processes on the top of the thoracic vertebrae—T3 to T9—as they emerge above the shoulder blades (scapulae).

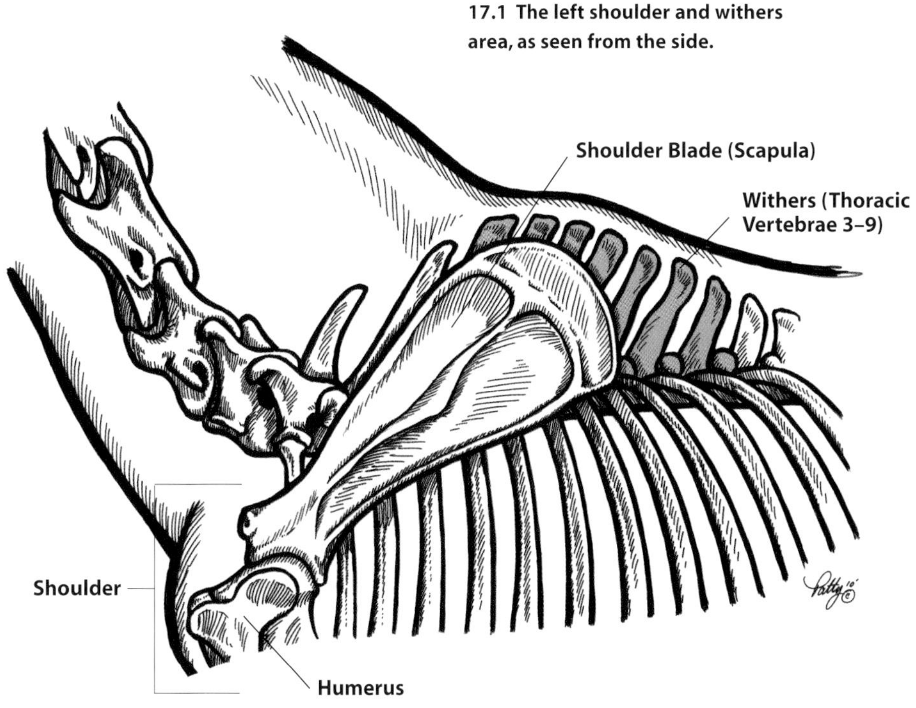

17.1 The left shoulder and withers area, as seen from the side.

RANGE OF MOTION: The withers have the same range of motion as the other thoracic vertebrae, but since they are partially covered by the shoulder blade (scapula), their movement is restricted in the standing horse. The normal range of motion for the withers of the standing horse is approximately one-half inch to each side. It is also very important that each vertebra is moving individually, and that they are not "stuck" to each other.

HOW TO

The withers are located just above the shoulder blades (fig. 17.2). Place the side of your hand along the wither bone you are checking, connecting your hand with as much of the vertebra as possible (fig. 17.3). Be sure the bottom of your hand does not rest on the shoulder blade. Do not use your thumbs, as they can create a pressure point and cause muscles to tense up. Use your free hand to hold the wither bone next to the one you are pushing to keep it still (fig. 17.4).

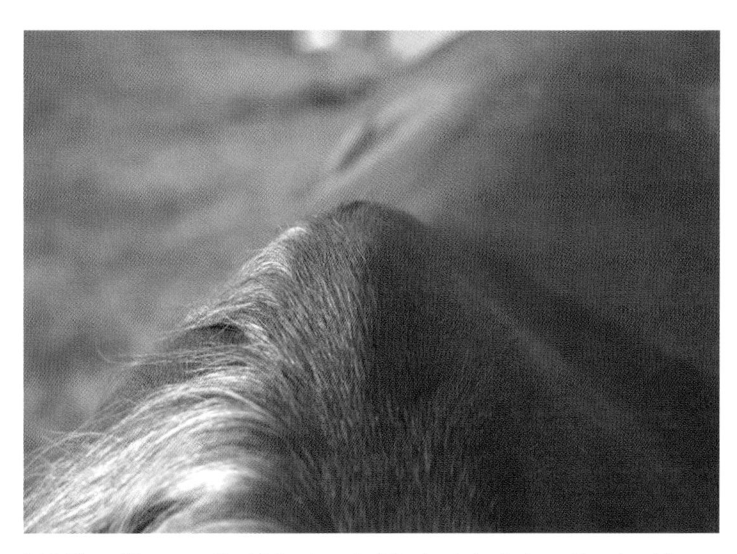

17.2 The withers are the highest part of the back, just above the shoulder blades. There are usually four to six separate bones (spinous processes) that you can feel along the withers area.

Gently push the wither bone to one side of the horse and release it to allow it to go back to center. Do this a few times to get the feel of its range of motion. Do not push the wither bone to the side and hold it there. This causes muscles to tighten and you will not be able to feel the wither bones' true range of motion. Be sure to check all the wither bones you can reach (the ones above the shoulder blades) and check them from both sides of the horse.

Mutton-Withered—Really?

Many people refer to horses with small withers as "mutton-withered." True "mutton-withered" horses have no withers whatsoever. They have no thoracic vertebrae (withers) protruding above the shoulder blades, just like sheep—hence the name! You should note that truly "mutton-withered" horses cannot be checked with this technique.

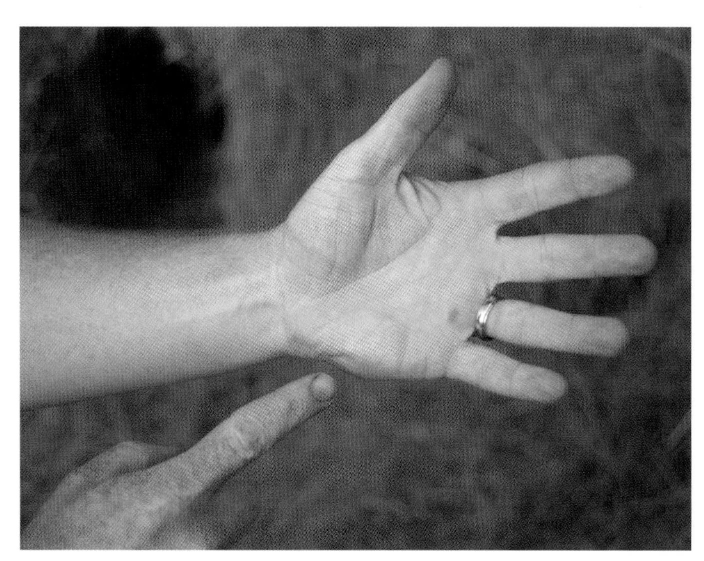

17.3 The side of the hand is indicated here.

Diagnosis

Normal wither vertebrae can move at least one-half inch to the left and to the right. If a wither bone cannot move in either direction, or only one direction, it is subluxated.

Summary: WITHERS

- When any of the wither bones cannot be moved, call chiropractor. Or, try some massage or another healing modality once or twice in the withers area to release them. If the wither bones remain "stuck," call chiropractor.
- When no indication of subluxation but symptoms remain, check for:
    - Subluxations at: shoulder, shoulder blade, ribs, sternum (pp. 69, 66, 117, 74)
    - Heel-pain syndrome
    - Ulcers
    - Saddle fit

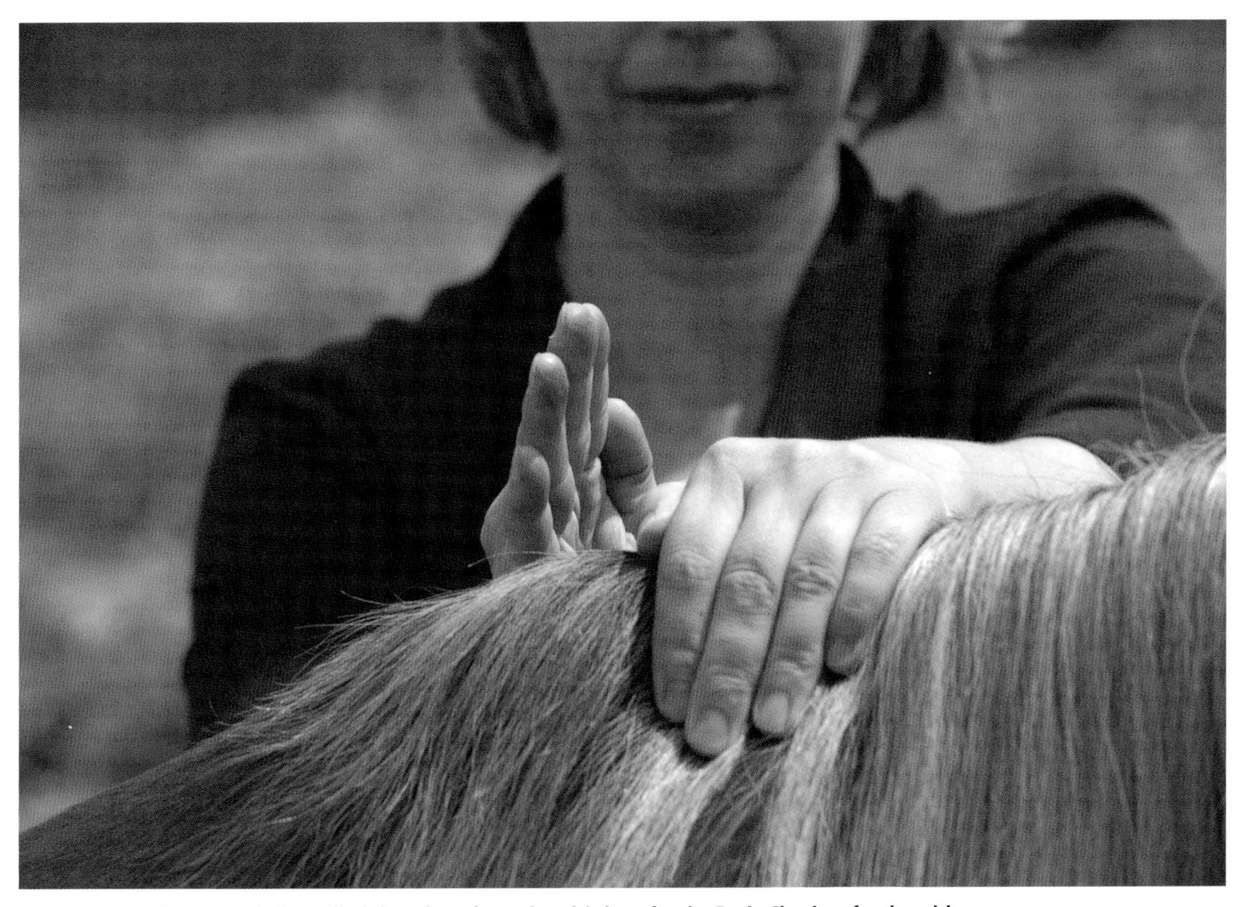

17.4 The side of your hand, also called the edge of your hand, is best for the Body Checkup for the withers.

BODY CHECKUP 18
THE THORACIC VERTEBRAE

Do you ever have that sneaking suspicion that something is just not right? I had been working on this Friesian/Thoroughbred cross named Chili for a few months. It seemed like his body would adjust well, and the horse and owner would be happy for a few weeks, but then things would unravel again. (I hate that!)

Chili's owner and I had gone over everything I could think of that might cause the adjustments to not hold well. We talked about nutrition, foot angles, saddle fit, and teeth floating. I quizzed her on falls, trauma, or crashes that might have happened in the past. We talked about behavior problems like cribbing; tongue-sucking; weaving; kicking the stall walls; or digging holes and lying down in them. But there was nothing.

I had to refocus. We did an adjustment and I asked her if I could come back in five days to recheck. When I came back, the areas with issues were the thoracic vertebrae, with some ribs out of adjustment, as well. Aha! These symptoms pointed to saddle fit as the culprit. Although I had already spoken with her about her saddle, I now asked her if I could see it. She reminded me that this was a "very expensive saddle that was custom fit to Chili," rather firmly implying that there was no need for me to check her saddle. I just said, "I bet it is gorgeous! I'd love to see it on him, if you don't mind."

She got her saddle out of its case and put it on Chili and…it was way too tight. Not at the shoulders where most people check, but in the gullet, which was too narrow in the thoracic spine area. This had caused Chili to hollow his back, interfering with his ability to develop a good topline. (It can also cause thoracic and rib subluxations.)

I find saddle fit to be a very common problem. Today I always check all the saddles a horse is ridden in on my first visit—even custom-made ones. I highly recommend Dr. Joyce Harman's saddle-fitting books and DVDs, so you can check your own saddles: *The Horse's Pain-Free Back and Saddle-Fit Book* and *The Western Horse' Pain-Free Back and Saddle-Fit Book*, and the DVDs *English Saddles* and *Western Saddles* (www.horseandriderbooks.com).

THORACIC VERTEBRAE CHALLENGE LEVEL 
Locating Anatomic Area: ★
Positioning of Horse or Handler: ★★
Subtle Range of Motion: ★★★
Complex Evaluation of Checkup: ★★

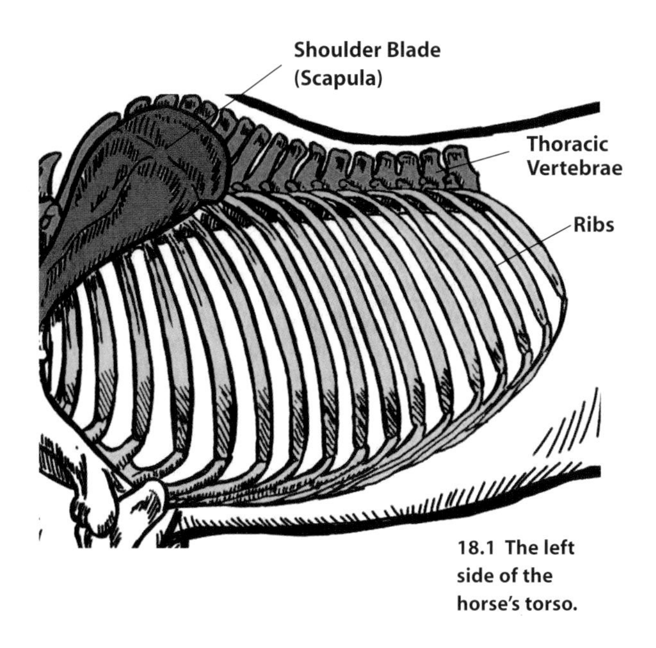

18.1 The left side of the horse's torso.

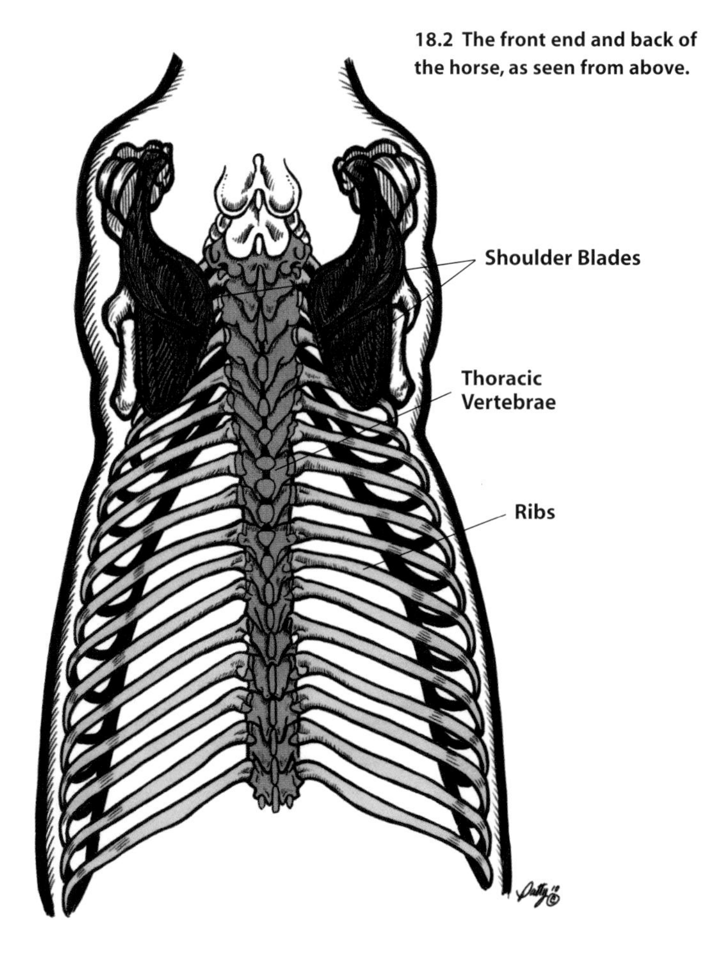

18.2 The front end and back of the horse, as seen from above.

Common Symptoms

BEHAVIOR OR PERFORMANCE SYMPTOMS

Very Common

- Horse feels stiff all over
- Reluctant to bend
- Difficulty using topline muscles properly
- Difficulty with collection and/or impulsion
- Cold-backed

Frequent

- Unable to stand still, especially when being mounted

Occasional

- Hypersensitivity to brushing
- Rolling excessively
- Crow-hopping or bucking
- Prefers to trot over other gaits

PHYSICAL SYMPTOMS: CURRENT OR PRIOR

- Back-sore
- Saddle-fit difficulties
- Rib subluxations, chronic
- Topline, difficult to develop
- Rider feels like one stirrup is long, but it isn't
- Rider feels crooked or saddle slips to one side
- Hind end doesn't naturally track up straight

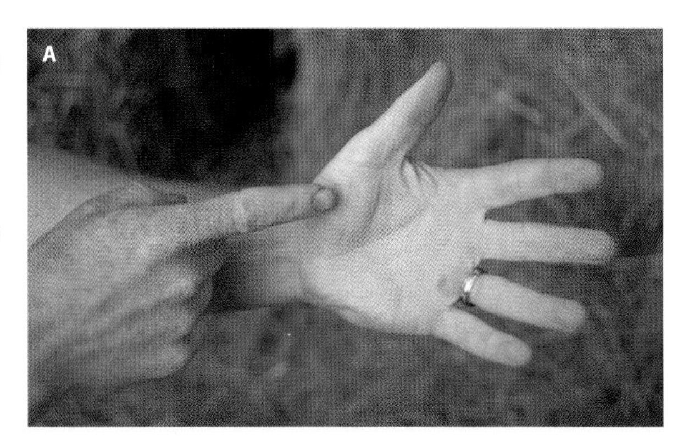

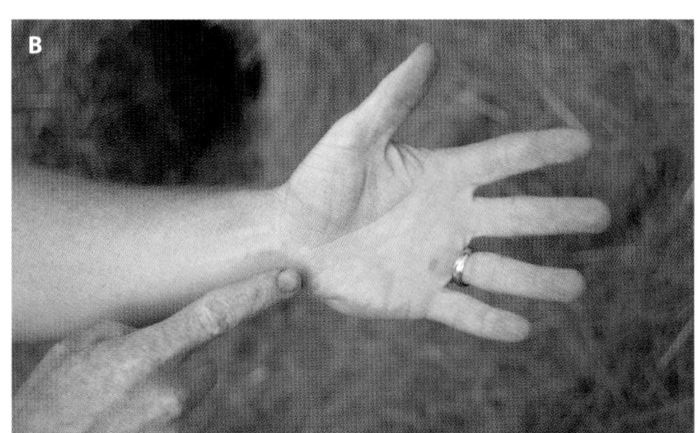

18.3 A & B The parts of the hand to use for checking the thoracic vertebrae: Photo A shows the thumb base, and B, the pisiform area.

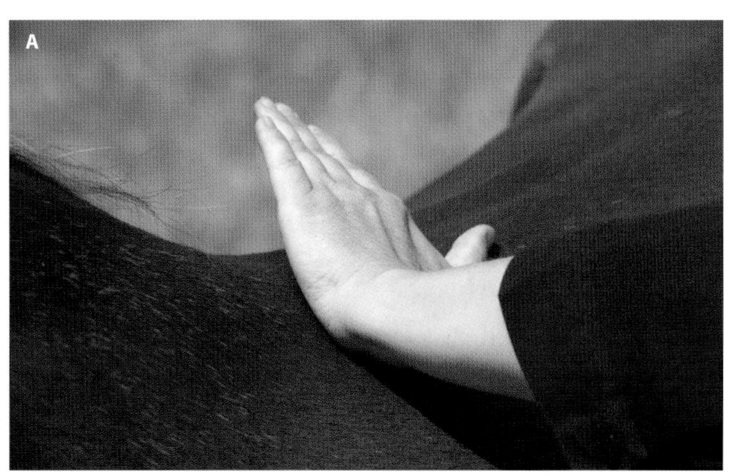

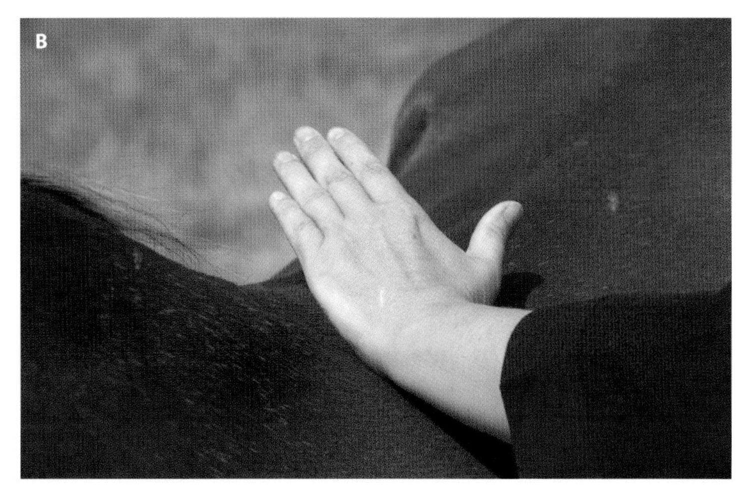

18.4 A & B I demonstrate this Body Checkup, using the base of my thumb in A, and the pisiform area of my hand in B.

Checkup Directions

FUNCTION: The function of the thoracic vertebrae is to form the spinal column of bones that protects the spinal cord. They also allow for flexibility in the back, both up and down and side to side.

RANGE OF MOTION: The thoracic range of motion is hard to describe: When you bend your back from side to side and feel the thoracic (upper back) vertebrae move, you get the idea. These thoracic vertebrae are attached to the ribs, and because of this, there is less flexibility in this area than in the lumbar (lower back) area. This is true in both you and your horse.

HOW TO

Use either the thumb base or the pisiform area of your hand for this Checkup (figs. 18.3 A & B). Choose the area most comfortable. (NOTE: This is the same as the Checkup for the lumbar vertebrae on

p. 122.) Checking one vertebra at a time, place your left hand (when working on the left side of the horse) about 1 inch below the thoracic spinous processes, which run along the midline of the horse's back (figs. 18.4 A & B).

Now, cup the fingers of your right hand around the top of the tail. Do not wrap your fingers under the tail—for your safety and the horse's comfort (fig. 18.5). Gently pull the tail toward you with your right hand while applying light pressure with your left hand to resist the bend of the horse's body toward you, and then let go of the tail

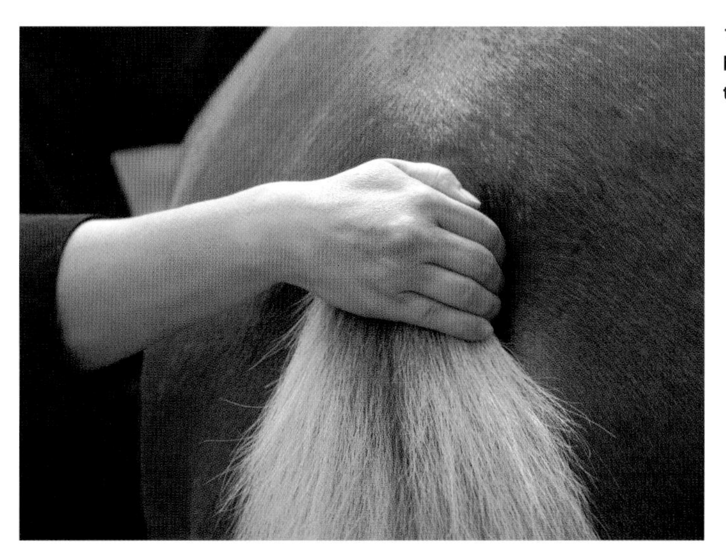

18.5 Place your free hand on the horse's tail, as shown here.

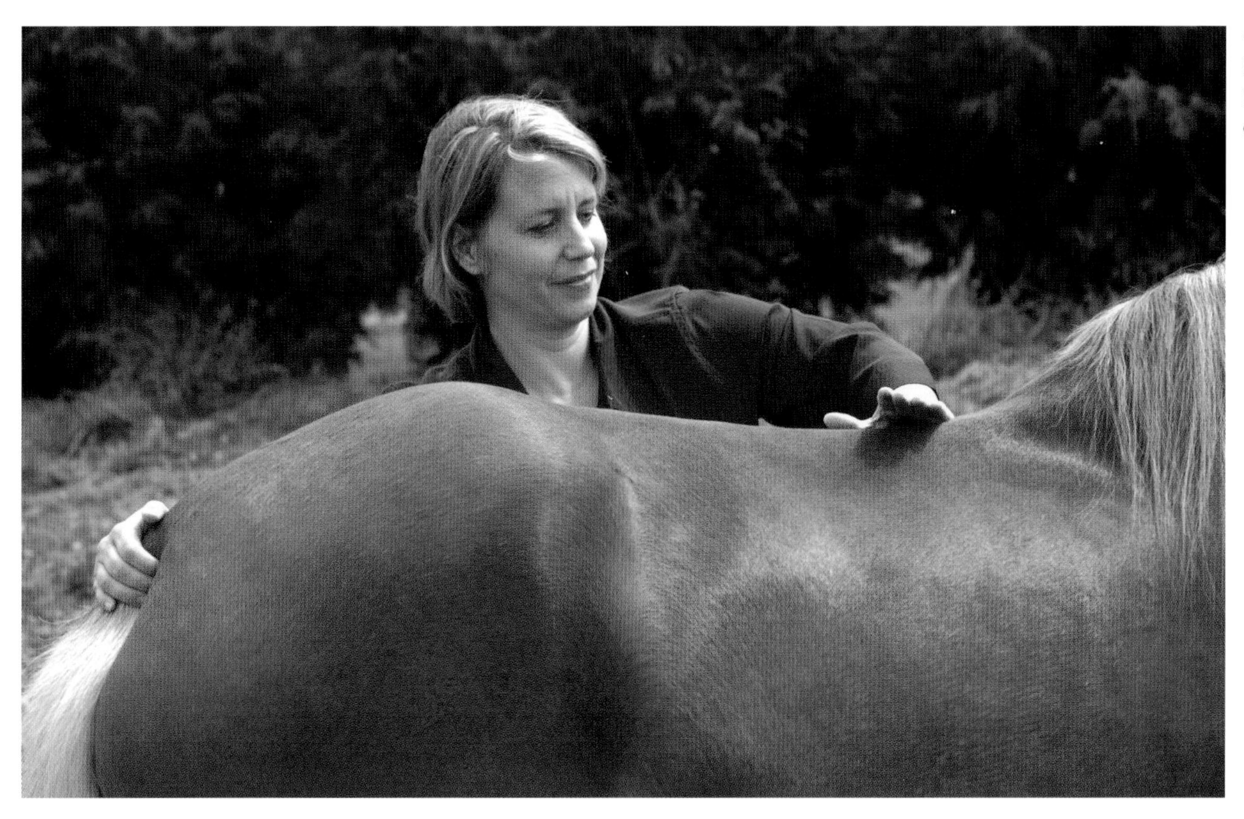

18.6 Here you can see both hand positions as I perform this Checkup on a thoracic vertebra.

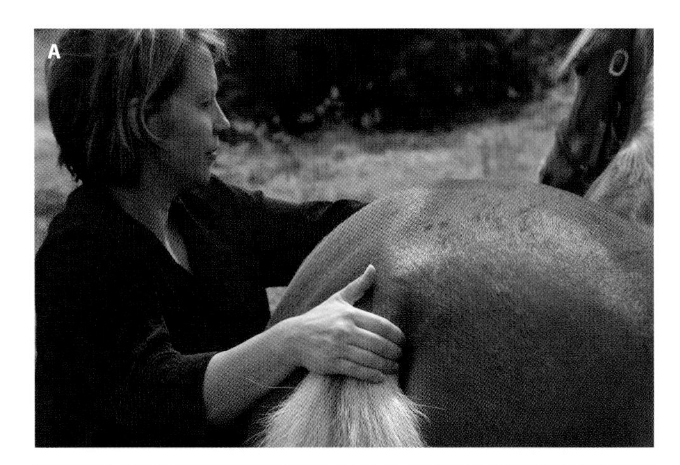

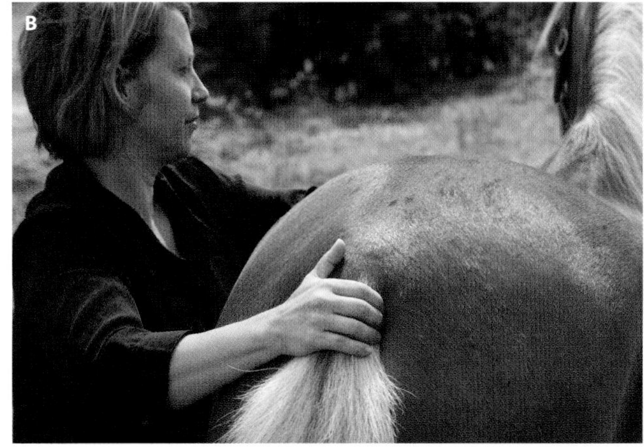

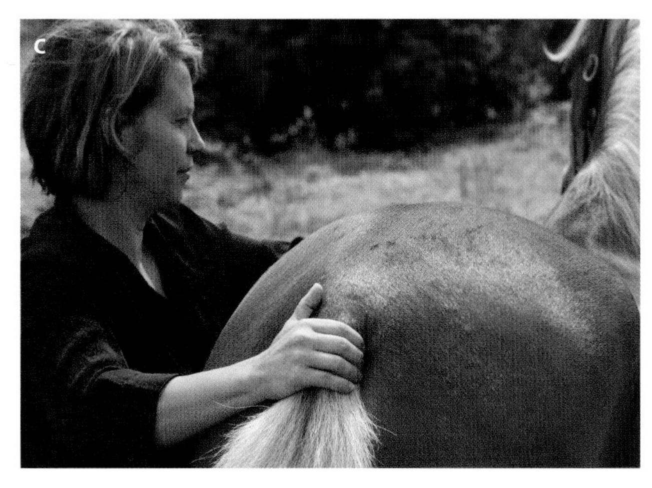

18.7 A–C This sequence shows the "wiggle" action you want in this Checkup, as seen from behind.

(fig. 18.6). Pull again. Let go again. As you get into a nice rhythm of pulling and letting go, you'll have a "wiggle" or "hula-hoop" action going with the horse's rear end (figs. 18.7 A–C). The wiggle will be primarily to the side you are working from. As this is happening, feel the thoracic vertebra under your hand moving. Then move your hand to the next thoracic vertebra's spinous process (you can check these in any order) and feel its movement.

Check each thoracic vertebra from T2 (the second thoracic vertebra), which is just in front of the withers, to T18, connected to the last rib. Check from both the left and right sides of the horse. The movement, or normal thoracic range of motion, can be difficult to quantify. In order to get practiced at this, I suggest you start by checking the lumbar area first (p. 122) to get a feel for this wiggle (it is more obvious there).

Diagnosis

When there are thoracic vertebrae that noticeably do not move as much as the others during the wiggle, there are most likely subluxations. If all of the thoracic vertebrae feel the same and very stiff, it's likely your horse is bracing against the movement to protect himself from rib, or another source of subluxation pain.

Summary: THORACIC VERTEBRAE

- When subluxations suspected, call chiropractor.
- When no indication of subluxation but symptoms remain, check for:
    - Subluxations at: ribs, lumbar vertebrae, withers (p. 117, 122, 108)
    - Saddle Fit

BODY CHECKUP 19
THE RIBS

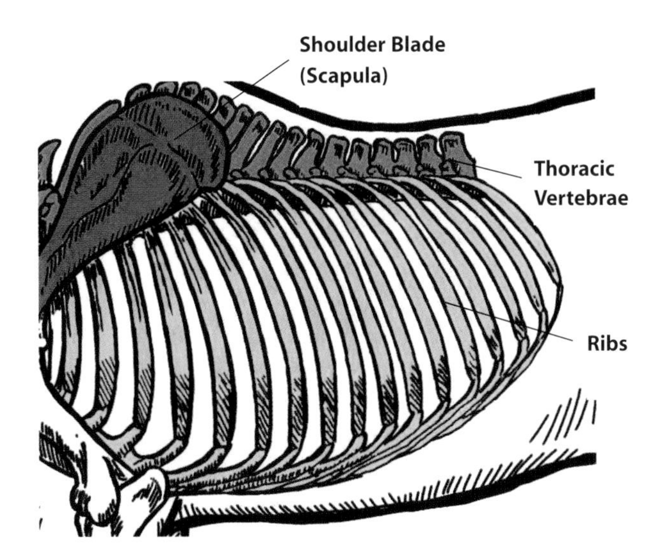

19.1 The horse has 18 ribs. The first rib through the seventh rib (approximately) are covered by the shoulder blade (scapula). Therefore, you check ribs 8 through 18 in this Checkup.

You would not believe how many horses have their ribs subluxated, or "out" as I tend to say. I know when I have a rib out. The first day, it really hurts, then it becomes just a dull ache.

I fell facedown while I was trying to learn to snowboard. I heard a pop and I was certain that I had cracked a rib. But then it didn't hurt—that is, unless I squeezed my shoulders in toward my chest, at which point it was as if someone had stuck a knife in my chest! When I pulled my shoulders back out, it stopped hurting completely.

I was sure I had fractured a rib and the spiky end of it was puncturing my lung. But since I could inhale and exhale just fine, I ruled that out. As you may have guessed, I had a subluxated rib.

The point of telling you this story is to explain why I have such admiration for a horse whose ribs are out. Like me, he probably doesn't hurt too much until a saddle is put on him, girthed up, and a rider is added—someone who wants the horse to move and bend through the rib cage. Yikes! I can understand why there are some horses out there that act like broncs, bucking like crazy whenever anyone gets on them. And, sadly, nobody understands why.

Won't it be great when someday horse pain is recognized as pain, and not bad behavior?

Common Symptoms

BEHAVIOR OR PERFORMANCE SYMPTOMS

Very Common

- Cold-backed
- Stiff, but may often warm up to perform acceptably

RIBS CHALLENGE LEVEL ☆☆☆
Locating Anatomic Area: ☆☆
Positioning of Horse or Handler: ☆
Subtle Range of Motion: ☆☆
Complex Evaluation of Checkup: ☆☆☆

- Difficulty bending in one or both directions
- Short-striding in front or rear
- Lack of front-end extension
- "Girthy"/"cinchy"
- Difficulty with collection and/or impulsion

Frequent

- Reluctance to stretch front end
- Shoulder has tightness, decreased range of motion, and is difficult to stretch
- Anything "weird" with the shoulder
- Hypersensitivity to brushing
- Difficulty picking up, maintaining, or changing leads
- Unable to stand still, especially when being mounted

Occasional

- Rolling excessively
- Crow-hopping or bucking
- Drops shoulder on turns
- Goes wide on turns
- Struggles with hind-end lateral work
- Shoulder muscles sore
- Tripping
- Prefers to trot over other gaits

PHYSICAL SYMPTOMS: CURRENT AND PRIOR

- Back-sore
- Rider feels crooked or saddle slips to one side
- Shortness of breath
- Troubles with saddle fit
- Inability to work ("exercise intolerance")
- Feet land toe first
- Foot is "clubby" or has a tendency to grow excess heel

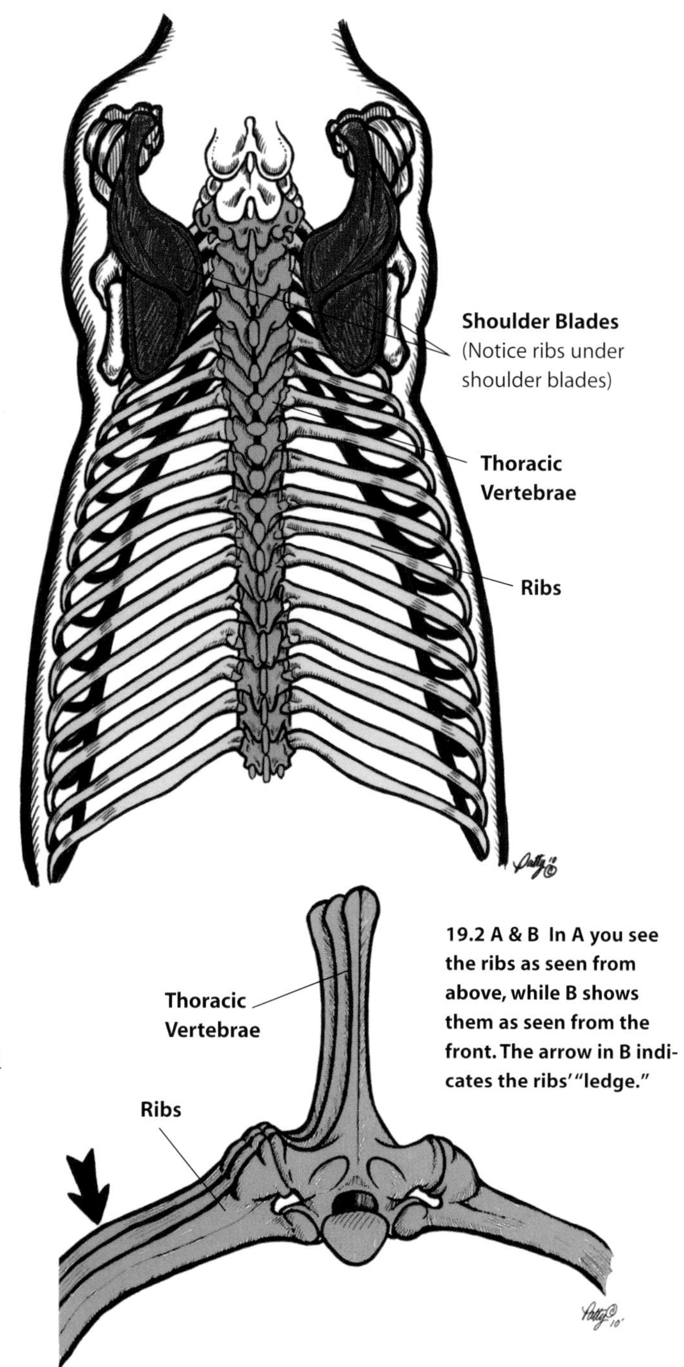

19.2 A & B In A you see the ribs as seen from above, while B shows them as seen from the front. The arrow in B indicates the ribs' "ledge."

Checkup Directions

FUNCTION: Besides being the bony protection for the thoracic cavity, the ribs allow for flexibility through the barrel of the horse.

RANGE OF MOTION: Due to the horse's anatomy, you are unable to check the true range of motion of the ribs. Instead, look for a light pain response (an "ouch") when the ribs are placed under pressure in a particular manner.

HOW TO

Check the ribs just past the shoulder blade all the way to the flank. These are attached to vertebrae T8 through T18. You'll be able to feel each individual rib's

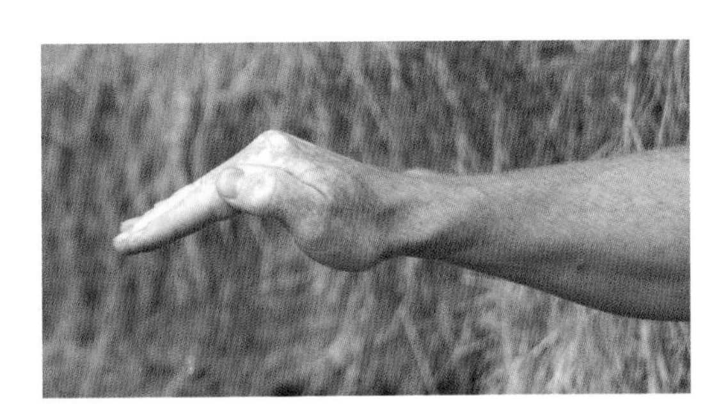

19.3 The hand position for finding the ribs' "ledge."

19.4 A–C Place your hand in the midline of the horse's back and slide it toward the barrel while pushing down. You will land on the ribs' "ledge."

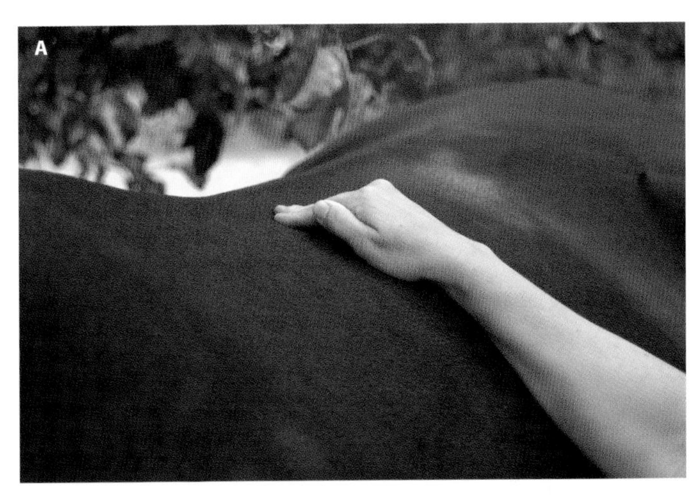

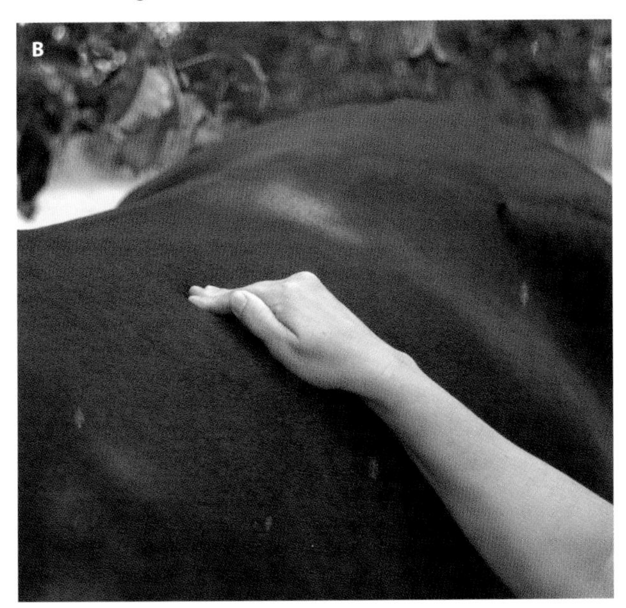

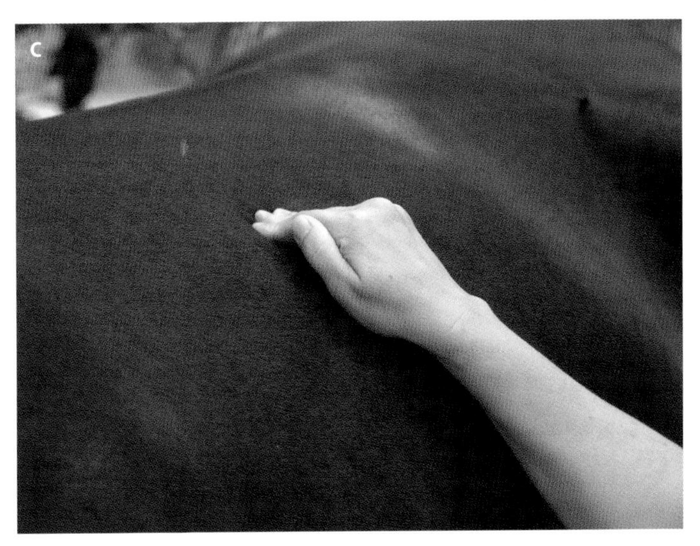

For ease of description, I use the term "rib head" in this Checkup, even though anatomically a rib's head is further in, nearer to the thoracic spinal processes.

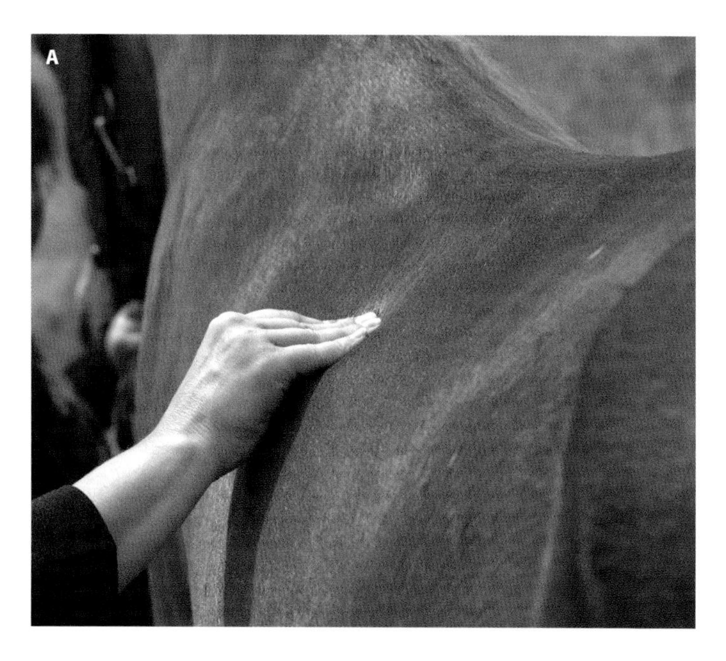

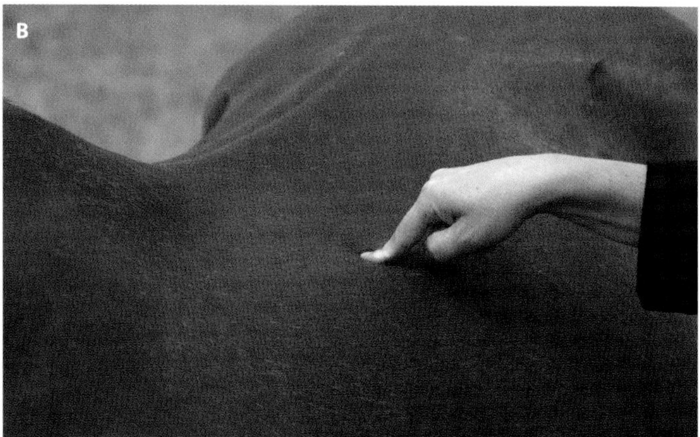

19.5 A & B In A, I have found the ribs' "ledge." In B, I press down vertically with my fingertip pad onto a rib "head." NOTE: While the finger itself is at an angle, the pressure is directly vertical.

"head" located beneath the spinal process as a "bump" along the ribs' "ledge." To locate this ledge, hold your hand with your fingers bent (fig. 19.3). Place it in the midline of the back and slide it toward the barrel while pushing down. You will land on the ribs' ledge when you push hard enough—but don't push too hard on a skinny horse (figs. 19.4 A–C).

If the horse is on the skinny side, you may feel another smaller ledge before the ribs' ledge. This first ledge is made up of the lateral processes of the thoracic vertebrae. The lateral processes project outward from the center of the spine about 7 inches. They end about one inch above the ribs' ledge. Again, the horse has to be pretty skinny (ribs almost visible) to feel this first ledge. You'll know when you've come to the ribs' ledge because, if you continue past it, your hands slide down onto the ribs themselves.

This ribs' ledge continues from the shoulder blade all the way to the flank. As you run your hand along it, you feel the subtle "bumps," which are each rib's "head." To do the Checkup, simply press down vertically on a rib's head with your fingertip(s) (figs. 19.5 A & B).

Be sure the pressure you apply is straight down vertically, not inward toward the horse. Also, use the pads of your fingertips, not the tips themselves. That would be the equivalent of poking the horse in the ribs—and he wouldn't like that!

Diagnosis

When there is a consistent, repeatable pain response (such as flinching, muscle spasm, tail switching, an irritated look), the rib is subluxated. NOTE: The pressure needed to check for rib subluxation is extremely individual. With some horses—for example, a typical Thoroughbred—you need to use the pressure that you would use to squeeze a firm peach. With another horse, such as a Warmblood, you need to use such firm pressure that you are using all the arm muscles you've got just to keep your wrist straight. Even with that much pressure, a Warmblood typically only gives a very tiny muscle twitch when a rib is subluxated. Any consistent pain response (however small) is a subluxated rib.

Checking for subluxated ribs can also be tricky because some horses hold their breath when you first start pressing around their ribs. Others start dancing around to avoid the exam. Start with a light pressure and only press as hard as you need to see a response. A non-subluxated rib will be unresponsive to full finger pressure (approximately as much finger pressure as you would need to make an indent on a tennis ball).

Summary: RIBS

- Rib subluxations are very common, so when pain is apparent, call chiropractor and have saddle fit checked because it is the most common cause of rib subluxations.
- When no indication of subluxation but symptoms remain, check for:
    - Subluxations at: thoracic vertebrae; withers; lumbar vertebrae; C7 (p. 112, 108, 122, 60)
    - Ulcers
    - Saddle fit

BODY CHECKUP 20

THE LUMBAR VERTEBRAE

A horse's hind footprints should track directly in line with his front footprints, and during movement, step into the space the forefeet have just left (fig. 20.1 A). When this happens correctly, it's called "tracking up." When both of the horse's hind prints are over to the same side—even an inch—and it is not due to rider aids (as in the haunches-in or haunches-out), there are likely subluxations causing the lumbar area to curve (figs. 20.1 B & C). I've seen a horse whose hind prints were over to the side by 12 inches! It made my own back hurt just watching that poor horse walk.

However, when both hind feet track to the inside or both track to the outside of the front prints, it does not necessarily indicate chiropractic difficulties (figs. 20.1 D & E).

Check your horse's hoofprints the next time you ride in a freshly raked arena…or on the beach!

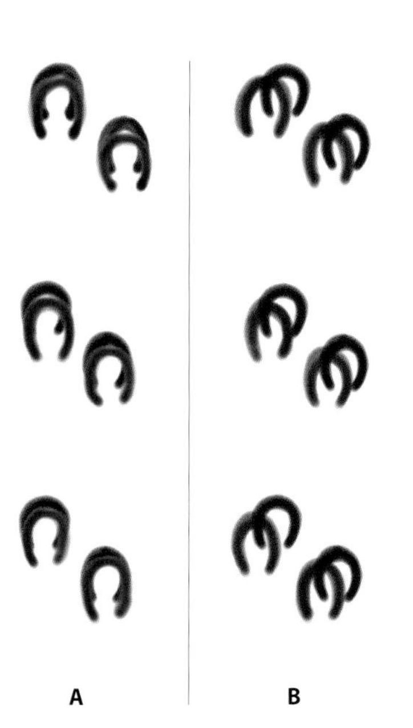

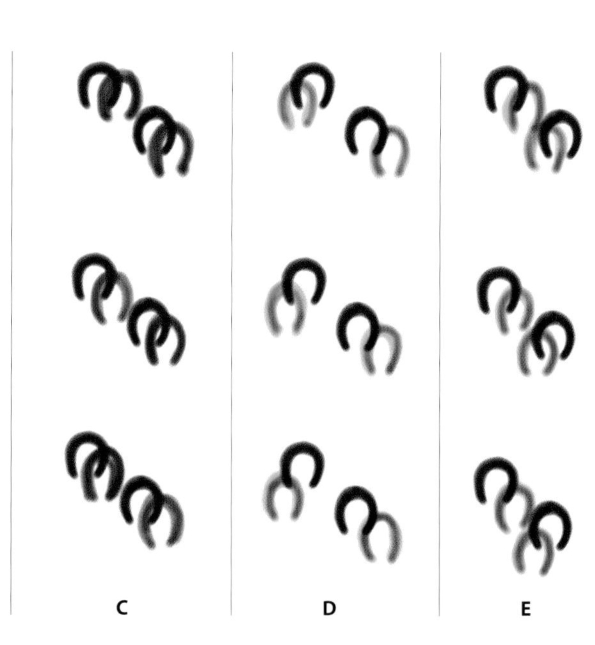

20.1 A–E Column A shows correct "tracking up." The hind feet are stepping directly forward into the prints of the front feet. Column B shows both hind feet tracking a few inches off to the left of the front feet, and column C shows them to the right. This is most likely caused by chiropractic subluxations. Column D shows both hind feet tracking to the outside of the front feet, and column E shows them tracking to the inside of the front feet. Both the latter cases are most likely *not* caused by chiropractic subluxation.

Common Symptoms

BEHAVIORAL OR PERFORMANCE SYMPTOMS

Very Common

- Difficulty with lateral bending
- Short-striding behind
- Difficulty with collection and/or impulsion
- Struggles with "long-and-low" work

Frequent

- Cold-backed
- Difficulty with gait transitions
- Difficulty picking up, maintaining, or changing leads
- Difficulty cantering/loping one or both directions
- Stiff body, may warm up to perform acceptably

Occasional

- Difficulty holding the hind feet up for the farrier
- Consistently resting one hind leg (either the same leg or alternating)
- Difficulty tracking straight
- Unable to stand still, especially when being mounted
- Hypersensitivity to brushing
- Rolling excessively
- Crow-hopping or bucking
- Rider sometimes feels like the horse "stepped in a hole"
- Rider sometimes feels the horse "dropped out from underneath" her
- Reluctant to go downhill
- Prefers to trot over other gaits
- Uneven hind-end takeoff when jumping
- Tail held to one side, either moving or at rest

PHYSICAL SYMPTOMS: CURRENT OR PRIOR

- Back-sore
- Tight lumbar muscles ("lumbar hump")
- Rider feels crooked or saddle slips to one side
- Hocks or stifles are sore or have other problems
- Stocking up in hind end
- Difficulty developing topline muscles
- Tail-clamping

LUMBAR VERTEBRAE CHALLENGE LEVEL 
Locating Anatomic Area: ☆
Positioning of Horse or Handler: ☆
Subtle Range of Motion: ☆☆☆
Complex Evaluation of Checkup: ☆☆

Checkup Directions

FUNCTION: The lumbar vertebrae are the most mobile in the horse's back. This is because they are not attached to the ribs like the thoracic vertebrae (p. 112). Because the lumbar vertebrae are the most mobile, they are called upon by the body to compensate for virtually any problem.

L6

The sixth lumbar vertebra (some horses have only five) is the last lumbar vertebra before the sacrum. It sits lower than the other vertebrae and is difficult to feel. It also has a more complicated range of motion due to its sacral connection. Consequently, checking the L6 vertebra has a five-star overall Challenge Level and is not covered in this book.

RANGE OF MOTION: To check lumbar motion, use the side-to-side movement of the hind end. As an example, bend yourself side to side through the waist, thus moving your lumbar (or lower back) vertebrae. The horse's hind end can easily move at least 6 inches to each side (measuring tail movement).

HOW TO

Place the side edge of your hand or the lower, fleshy part of your thumb—whichever is more comfortable—alongside the lumbar vertebra you are checking (see figs. 18.4 A & B, p. 114). Place it approximately one-half to one inch away from the midline of the back, while cupping your other hand over the base of the tail head. Be careful not to get your fingers under the tail (figs. 20.4 A & B).

Because the lumbar area compensates, or "picks up the slack" for almost every musculoskeletal problem a horse can have, it should be checked for every issue.

Gently pull the tail toward you while keeping your lumbar hand still. This hand: 1) keeps the horse from stepping toward you as you pull the tail and 2) feels the motion of the lumbar vertebra as it flexes under your hand.

As soon as the horse's hind end has moved toward you as far as it can easily go, release it. If you hold it in a flexed position, new muscles will engage and you will not be testing the lumbar vertebra. Pull and release again a few times. As you pull and release, the horse's hind end should do a "wiggle" or "hula-hoop" movement (see figs. 18.7 A–C, p. 116). Do this on the first five lumbar vertebra, L1 through L5, and check from both sides of the horse.

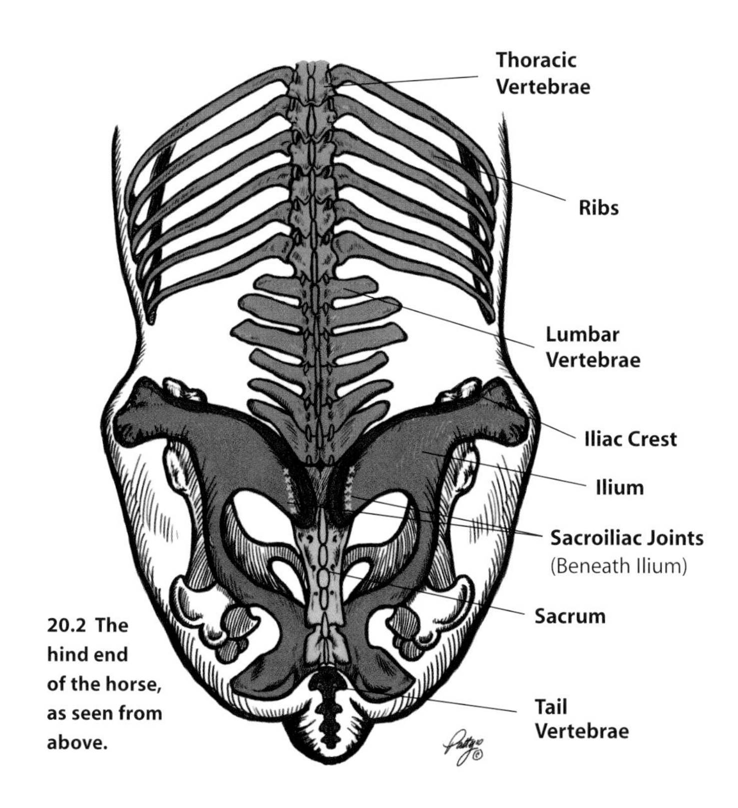

20.2 The hind end of the horse, as seen from above.

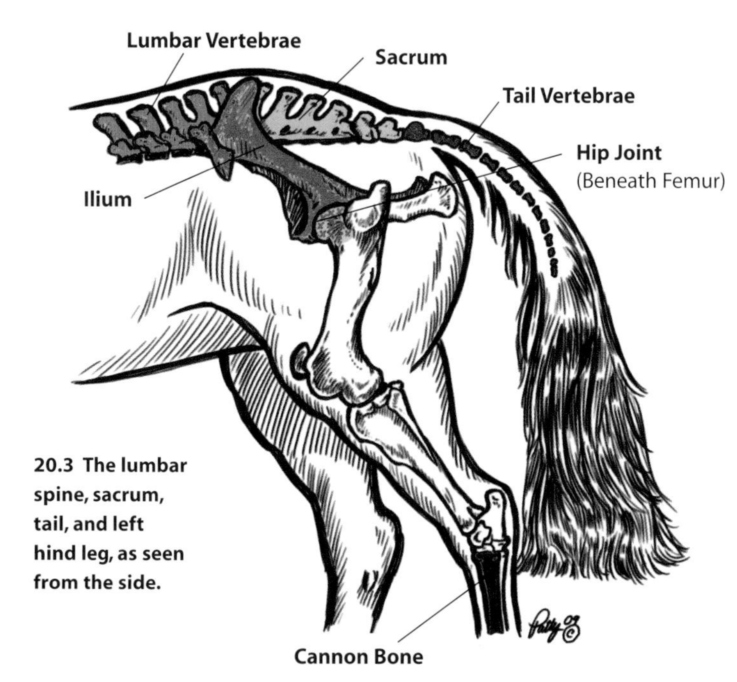

20.3 The lumbar spine, sacrum, tail, and left hind leg, as seen from the side.

Diagnosis

If any of the lumbar vertebrae do not move as well as the others, or if an entire side of the lumbar vertebrae does not move as well when compared to the other side, then you most likely have chiropractic subluxations. Occasionally the lumbar vertebrae can be "locked up" equally on both sides. You'll need experience with a number of horses to determine when this is the case.

Summary: LUMBAR VERTEBRAE

- When subluxations apparent, call chiropractor.
- When no indication of subluxation but symptoms remain, check for:
    - Subluxations at: ribs; sacroiliac joint; thoracic vertebrae; sacrum; intertransverse joint (pp. 117, 134, 112, 130, 126)
    - Hock issues
    - Stifle issues
    - Vitamin and/or mineral deficiency
    - Saddle fit

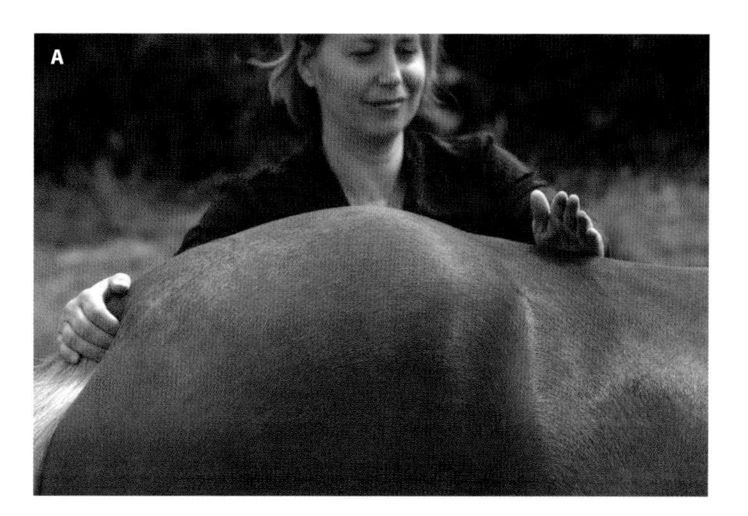

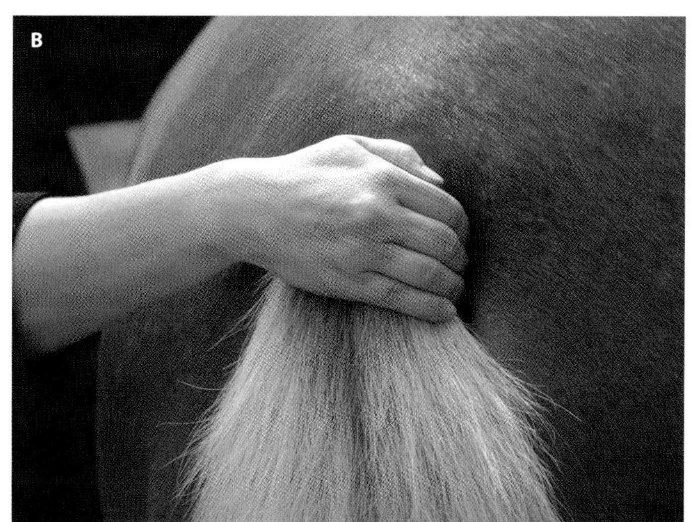

20.4 A & B Here, I demonstrate checking the lumbar vertebrae using the side edge of my hand placed one inch away from the midline of the spine, while holding the tail correctly.

BODY CHECKUP 21
THE INTERTRANSVERSE JOINT

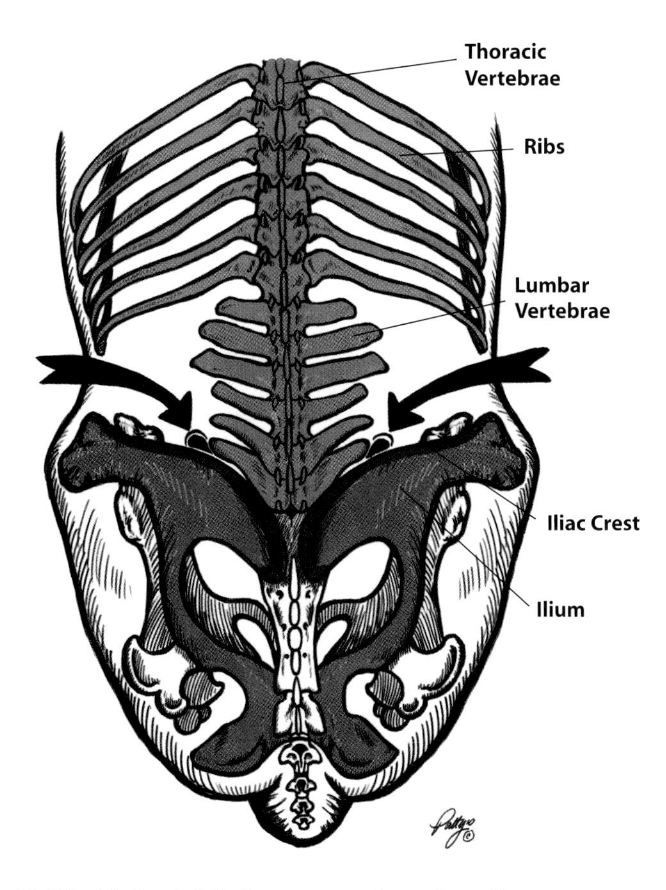

21.1 The hind end of the horse, as seen from above. The intertransverse joint area—indicated by the arrows—is represented by the black "teardrop" shapes.

One afternoon I was working in a barn and this horse owner I know, Debbie, asked me to recheck her nine-year-old Appaloosa mare named Baby.

I had adjusted Baby one week earlier, but Debbie had seen her take a bad slip. She hadn't actually fallen down but had managed to keep her feet during her slide through the mud. So, I wasn't expecting to find many subluxations, but was surprised when I found them in her left lumbar, left sacroiliac, sacrum, left hip, and the intertransverse joint. Despite all of these issues, my intuition told me that all was not as it seemed: She was acting extremely sensitive, particularly for such a tough Appy mare.

I rechecked all the subluxations, looking to find which one was causing the most pain. It turned out to be the intertransverse joint. So I adjusted that one first. Then I started to look for the next most sensitive area to adjust, but couldn't find one…because suddenly they were all gone!

This was a remarkable example of where the primary subluxation causes so much discomfort and

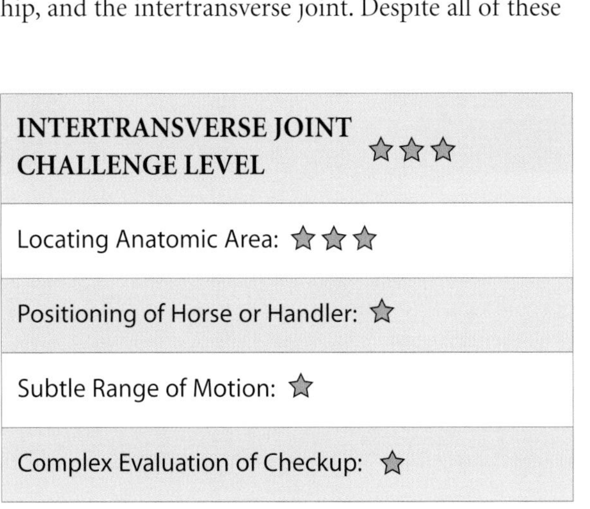

INTERTRANSVERSE JOINT CHALLENGE LEVEL ★★★
Locating Anatomic Area: ★★★
Positioning of Horse or Handler: ★
Subtle Range of Motion: ★
Complex Evaluation of Checkup: ★

stress that multiple other areas, called secondary subluxations, are pulled into misalignment in order to relieve stress on the first one. When the primary cause is fixed, all the others (in Baby's case) were able to fix themselves.

In a more chronic case, secondary subluxations may need help correcting themselves. In any event, the primary one needs to be corrected first, whenever possible.

Common Symptoms

BEHAVIORAL OR PERFORMANCE SYMPTOMS

*Very Common**

- Rests one hind leg or the other

*Frequent**

- Struggles with hind-end lateral work

Occasional

- Difficulty tracking straight
- Difficult to shoe
- Crow-hopping
- Short-striding behind

(NOTE: It is rare to see the intertransverse subluxated alone. These very common and frequent symptoms typically occur when the sacroiliac joint—p. 134—is also subluxated.)*

PHYSICAL SYMPTOMS: CURRENT OR PRIOR

- Pelvic subluxations (sacrum, sacroiliac, hip), recurring
- Lumbar subluxations, recurring

Checkup Directions

FUNCTION: The intertransverse joint is really a "pseudo" joint. If you look it up in a horse anatomy book, you probably will not find it. However, since it acts like a joint and adjusts like a joint, I will treat it as a joint.

The intertransverse functions as a miniature, partial ball-and-socket joint in between the last lumbar vertebra (L6) and the pelvis near the point of the hip. It supports and enhances the flexibility of the lumbar-to-pelvis connection.

RANGE OF MOTION: The intertransverse joint moves in all directions. In the standing horse, however, you are unable to evaluate its entire range of motion. Instead, look for a pain response to direct downward pressure, which indicates a subluxation of this joint.

HOW TO

A tricky part of checking the intertransverse joint is locating it. There are only muscular landmarks, and these may well be covered in a fat layer. It lies one-half to 2 inches in front of the center of the diagonal line connecting the point of the hip (tuber coxae) to the peak of the hind end (tuber sacrale) (fig. 21.2).

Feel for a small area approximately one-half to 1 inch at its greatest diameter. As you run your hand over the area, this point will feel like a bruise on a peach. Once found,

Acupuncture Point

Keep in mind the intertransverse area is also an acupuncture point often used for reproductive issues. If your mare has difficult heat cycles, this point may have a pain response unrelated to chiropractic subluxations.

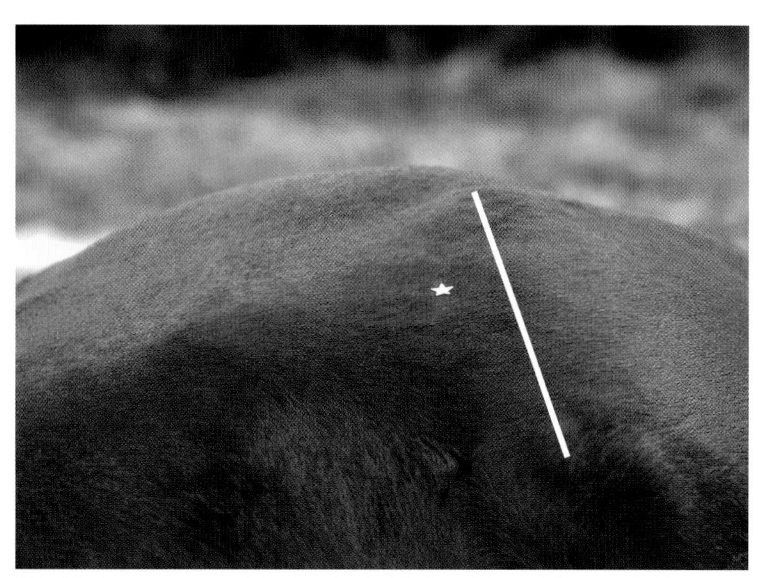

21.2 The intertransverse joint (marked with the white star) lies one-half to 2 inches in front of the center of the diagonal line connecting the point of the hip to the peak of the hind end.

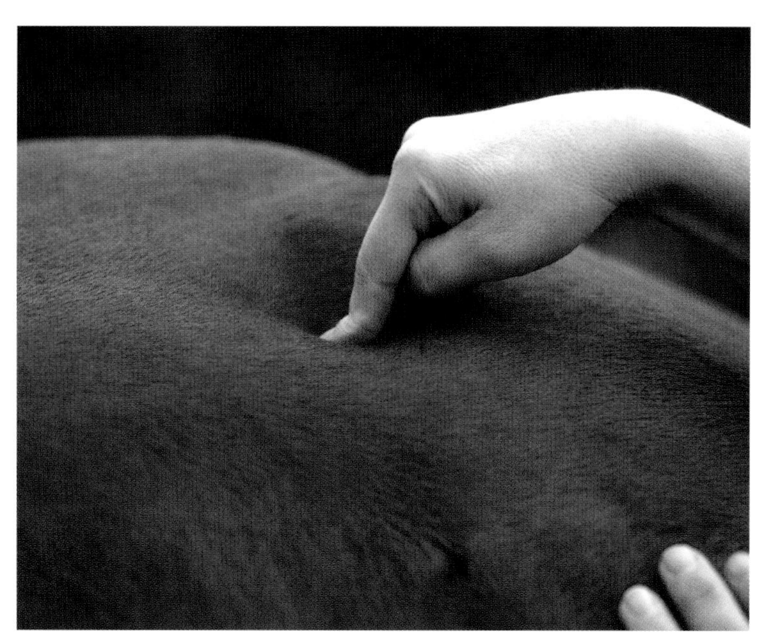

21.3 In this Checkup, I push down vertically on the intertransverse area. NOTE: The horse's hind end is to the right of this photo.

simply push down directly vertically with one finger (fig. 21.3).

Diagnosis

You should be able to push down until the muscle no longer "gives" without the horse flinching or tensing his muscles. This distance is approximately 1 inch. If there is consistent flinching as you push down, the intertransverse is subluxated.

Summary: INTERTRANSVERSE JOINT

- This area can be a "trigger point" for sore muscles, which is why the analysis of this Checkup is a bit tricky. If you have a sensitive intertransverse joint, no other sore muscles, and no mare cycling issues, then it is most likely subluxated—call the chiropractor.
- If your horse has sore muscles and/or mare-cycling issues, even if the intertransverse joint is subluxated, it is most likely due to other causes—resolve those first.
- When no indication of subluxation but symptoms remain, check for:
    - Subluxations at: lumbar vertebrae; sacrum; sacroiliac joint; hip (pp. 122, 130, 134, 137)
    - Hock issues
    - Stifle issues
    - Hoof-wall imbalance
    - Saddle fit

Section 4

THE HIND END BODY CHECKUPS

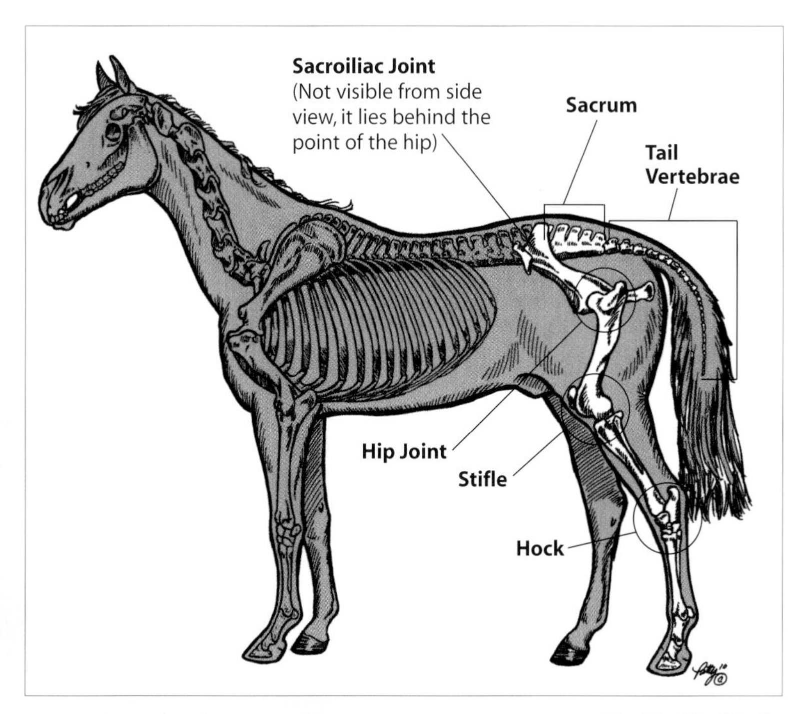

The Hind End Body Checkup areas

Hind End Problems: General Symptoms

- More comfortable with one lead than the other
- Difficulty picking up, maintaining, or changing leads
- Prefers to trot, rather than canter/lope or walk
- Rider feels like the horse "stepped in a hole"
- Rider feels the hind end "drop out from under her"
- Uneven hind-end takeoff when jumping, possibly creating twist through lumbar area
- Difficulty with collection or impulsion
- Unable to stand still, particularly when being mounted
- Crow-hopping
- Cold-backed
- Short-striding behind
- Standing with a hind leg turned out to the side
- Reluctance to jump
- Reluctance to do tight turns
- Holds tail to one side, either when moving or at rest
- Clamps tail when it is touched

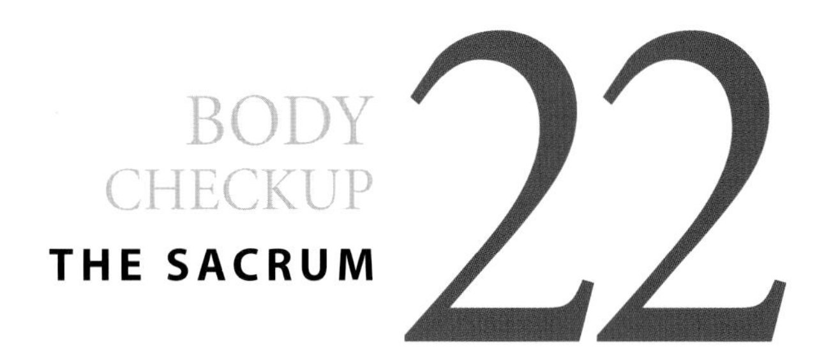

There are very few things in chiropractic treatment that are absolutely certain. Both lameness and/or behavior can give you clues to the general area of subluxation. However, there is one behavioral sign that is an absolute: swapping out leads behind. This is when 1) a horse has difficulty picking up a lead in the hind end only, and 2) a horse can pick up the correct lead in the hind end but soon "swaps it out" for the incorrect lead.

This *always* indicates the sacrum is subluxated. The horse may have other subluxations and the sacrum may not even be the primary problem, but it is definitely involved when lead-swapping is observed.

SACRUM CHALLENGE LEVEL ☆☆☆
Locating Anatomic Area: ☆☆
Positioning of Person or Horse: ☆
Subtle Range of Motion: ☆☆☆
Complex Evaluation of Checkup: ☆☆☆

Common Symptoms

BEHAVIORAL OR PERFORMANCE SYMPTOMS

Very Common

- Cross-cantering (different leads in front and behind)
- Difficulty picking up, maintaining, or changing leads
- Swapping out leads behind

Frequent

- Difficulty with collection or impulsion
- Stiff in hind end
- Struggles with hind-end lateral work
- Difficulty with gait transitions

Occasional

- Short-striding behind
- Crow-hopping
- Reluctance to jump
- Almost always rests one hind leg when standing
- Struggles with "long-and-low" work
- Makes life difficult for the farrier, especially hind end
- Hind end does not naturally track up straight
- Prefers to trot over other gaits
- Uneven takeoff when jumping

PHYSICAL SYMPTOMS: CURRENT OR PRIOR

- Phantom lameness behind
- Lumbar problems, chronic
- Tail-clamping
- Tail held to one side
- Gluteal muscles, consistent discomfort with massage

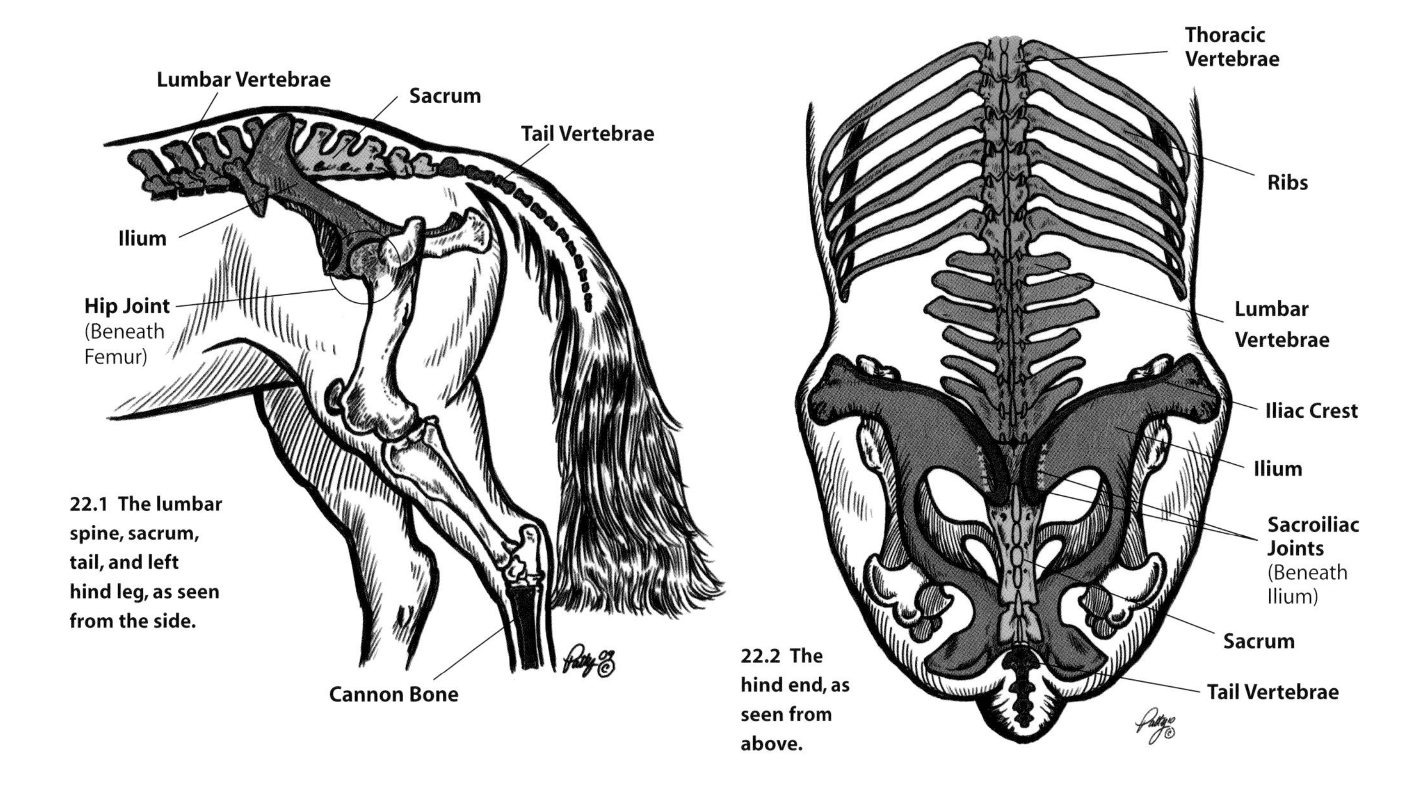

22.1 The lumbar spine, sacrum, tail, and left hind leg, as seen from the side.

22.2 The hind end, as seen from above.

Checkup Directions

FUNCTION: The sacrum is one of the two anchor points for the dura mater of the spinal cord. (The other is the atlas—see p. 44.) The spinal cord ends at the sacrum. Nerves branch out through spaces in the sacrum and continue down the legs. Because so many nerves are involved in the sacrum, its chiropractic alignment is very important for hind-end function.

RANGE OF MOTION: The sacrum connects to the pelvis via the sacroiliac joint, as well as to the lumbar area via the last lumbar vertebra (L6 or L5). The sacrum moves in a figure-eight pattern as the horse walks. For the sacrum Checkup in the standing horse, look for a small pain response to sideways pressure. The sacrum has five vertebrae in it. In the young horse these vertebrae move separately. In the mature horse, these five vertebrae have fused together to make the sacrum a functional "square" (see below).

HOW TO

The sacrum follows the lumbar vertebrae and is located at the highest point of the hind end to a few inches in front of the tail (fig. 22.3). If you imagine the right and left sides of the sacrum connected at the top and bottom, you get the idea that the sacrum is basically a square. When you do the sacrum Checkup, you are looking for any pain response to pressure

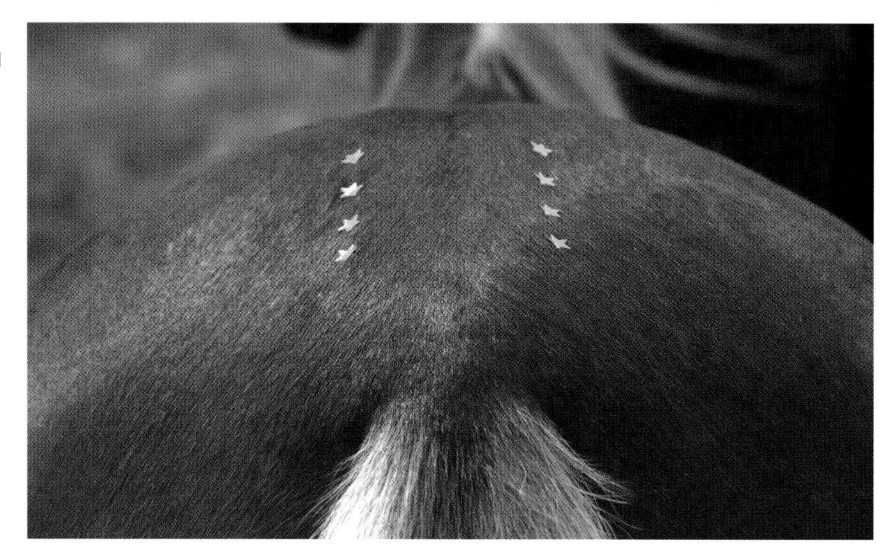

22.3 Here, the sacrum is outlined by green stars.

Place one hand over the bottom half of the sacrum. Cup your hand a bit to enable your finger pads to lightly "grab" the far edge of the sacrum. The base of your other hand will be applying stabilizing pressure to the other edge of the sacrum. With both of your hands applying pressure, the horse won't think you want him to step toward you (figs. 22.4 A & B). When your hands are in position, use the fingertips of the hand closest to the tail to pull the sacrum toward you. Use the same amount of pull

along the sides of the square. The "top" half of the sacrum is the half closest to the highest part of the hind end. The "bottom" half of the sacrum is the half closest to the tail. The reason for dividing the sacrum into "halves" is because most people can comfortably put both hands on the sacrum and cover it completely.

22.4 A & B In this Checkup one hand (here, my right) pulls the bottom half of the sacrum while the other (my left) applies light, stabilizing pressure to the top half. In B, the photo is angled to show the "grab" of the finger pads.

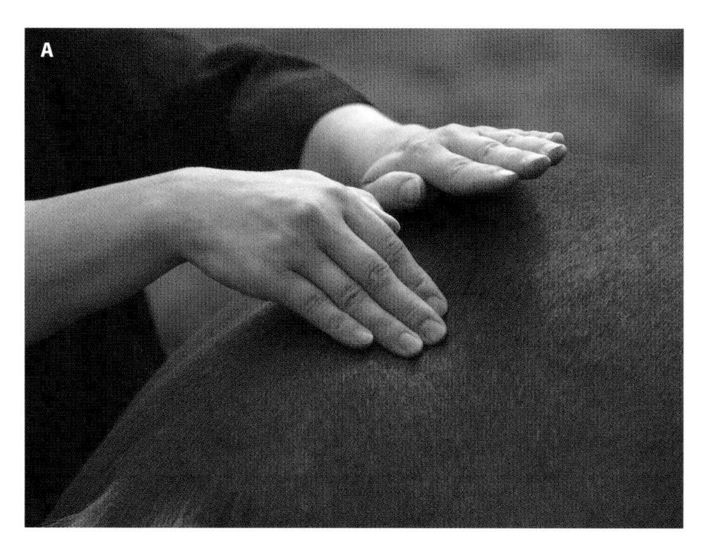

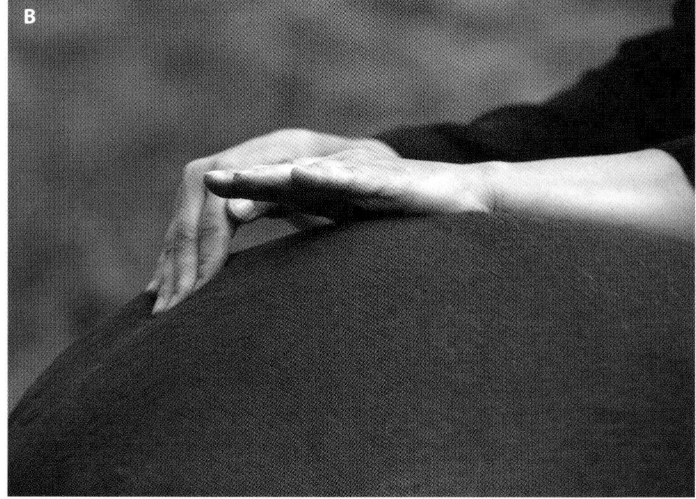

as you would to open a heavy screen door.

When using your fingertips, it is important not to use "poking" fingers, which make the horse flinch in pain. Use the flat pads of your fingers and pull, looking for muscles to flinch either in the gluteal (hind-end) or lumbar areas, or both.

Switch your hand positioning so that you pull the front half of the sacrum toward you while stabilizing with the base of your other hand (fig. 27.5). Be sure to perform the Checkup from both sides of the horse.

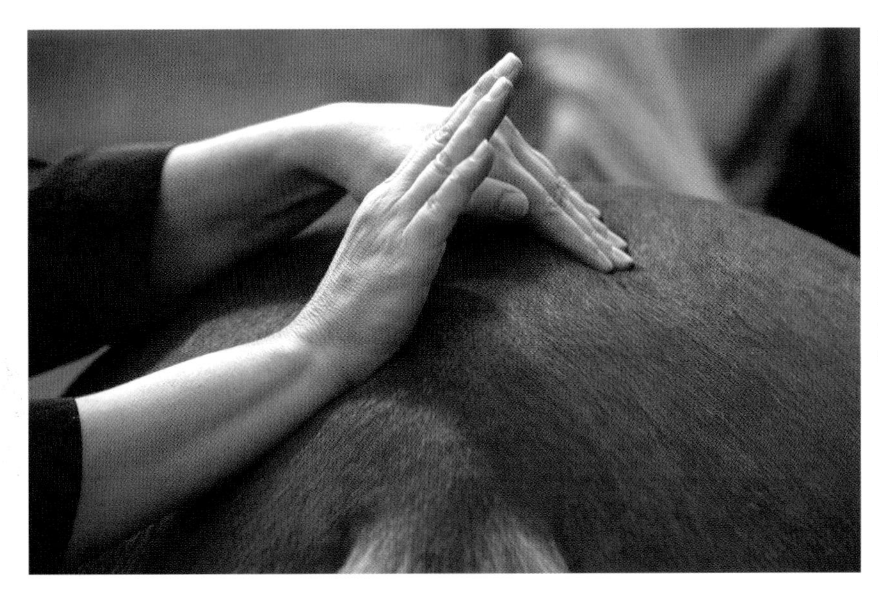

22.5 Here, my hand positions have switched: The left hand is now pulling the top half of the sacrum while the right hand applies light stabilizing pressure with the base of the hand to the bottom half of the sacrum.

Diagnosis

Any consistent muscle flinching in response to pulling the sacrum indicates sacral subluxation. The sacrum is relatively easy to examine for subluxation, because it either hurts or it doesn't. However, be aware that a sacrum subluxation can often be secondary to sacroiliac (SI), lumbar, tail, or hip subluxations, so check them, too. In addition, if you have a sacrum that keeps subluxating, you may have a pelvic symphysis (similar to the pubic bone) subluxation that is causing it. You'll need a certified chiropractor to diagnose this.

Summary: SACRUM

- When subluxations suspected, call chiropractor. NOTE: Recurrent sacral subluxations are frequently caused by some physical problem, such as hock or stifle issues. If your horse has recurrent sacral subluxations, it is wise to call your veterinarian.
- When no indication of subluxation but symptoms remain, check for:
  - Subluxations at: hock; stifle; sacroiliac joint; lumbar vertebrae; ribs; thoracic vertebrae; hip joint; tail vertebrae (pp. 145, 141, 134, 122, 117, 112, 137, 149)
  - Hoof-wall imbalance
  - Hock problems
  - Stifle problems
  - Vitamin and/or mineral deficiency

BODY CHECKUP 23 THE SACROILIAC JOINT

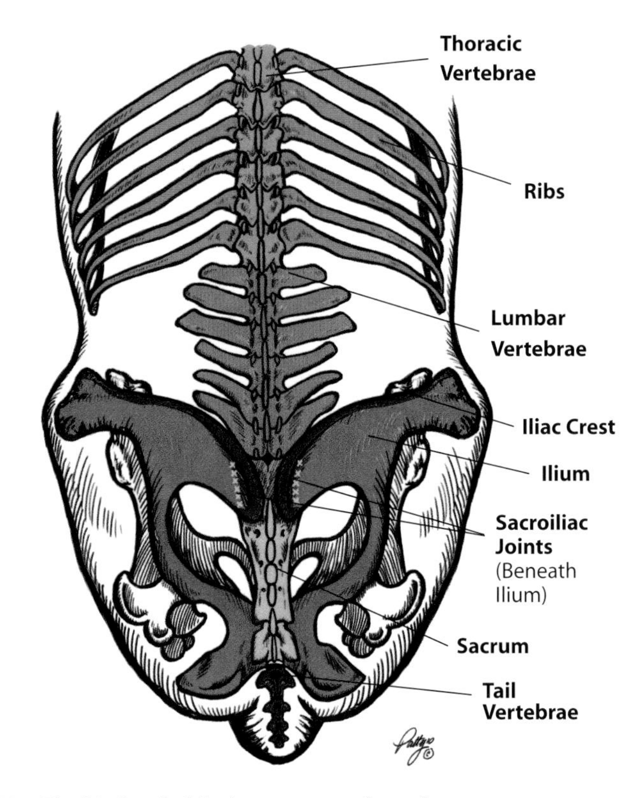

23.1 The hind end of the horse, as seen from above.

Two confusing terms are "lumbar hump" and "hunter's bump." A lumbar hump involves only the lumbar (lower back) area. It occurs when the lumbar muscles overtighten to compensate for problems elsewhere, and cause the lumbar area to "hump up." You can see this when viewed from the side. Very rarely, a horse may be born with a "lumbar hump" as a characteristic of his conformation.

A hunter's bump, if present, is located over one (rarely both) sacroiliac joints, and is most apparent when viewed from the rear. One sacroiliac joint will be noticeably higher than the other, perhaps as much as 2 inches. The height discrepancy is due to an increased growth of muscles and ligaments, as well as additional bone growth in the long-term case. The increase in muscle, ligament, and bone happens when the sacroiliac joint is subluxated and cannot function normally. This is most commonly seen in hunters and jumpers, especially those that have jumped for years using uneven propulsive force off their hind legs.

Lumbar humps and hunter's bumps can be seen in any type and breed of horse and both are very treatable with chiropractic and/or other healing modalities.

SACROILIAC JOINT CHALLENGE LEVEL ☆☆☆
Locating Anatomic Area: ☆☆
Positioning of Person or Horse: ☆
Subtle Range of Motion: ☆☆☆
Complex Evaluation of Checkup: ☆☆☆

Common Symptoms

BEHAVIORAL OR PERFORMANCE SYMPTOMS

Very Common

- More comfortable with one lead than another
- Difficulty picking up, maintaining, or changing leads
- Difficulty with collection or impulsion

Frequent

- Short-striding behind
- Struggles with hind-end lateral work
- Hind-end stiffness

Occasional

- Preferring to trot, rather than canter/lope or walk
- Rider feels like the horse "stepped in a hole"
- Rider feels the hind end "drop out from under her"
- Uneven hind-end takeoff when jumping
- Unable to stand still, particularly when being mounted
- Crow-hopping
- Cold-backed
- Makes life difficult for farrier, especially with hind end
- Almost always resting one hind foot
- Hind end does not naturally track up straight
- "Phantom" lameness in hind end

PHYSICAL SYMPTOMS: CURRENT OR PRIOR

- Hock soreness, history of
- Stocking up in hind end
- Lumbar subluxations, recurrent
- Sore gluteal muscles
- Rider feels crooked or saddle slips to one side

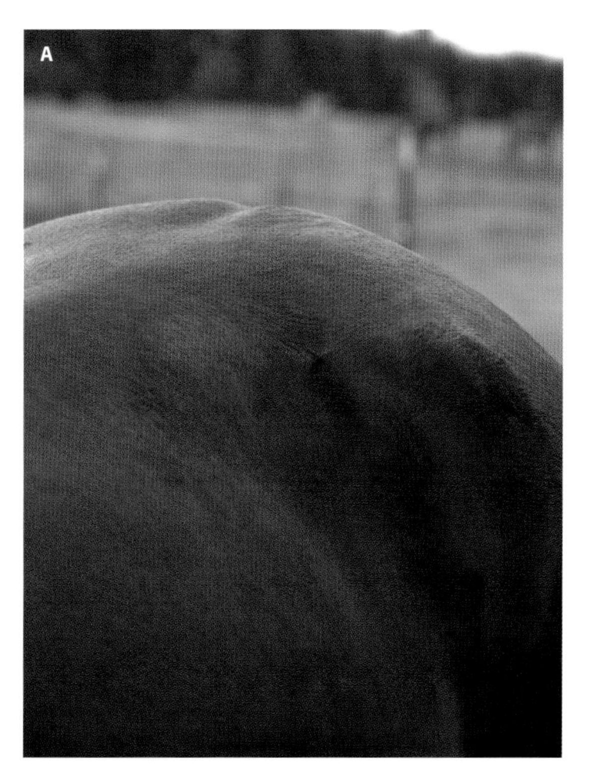

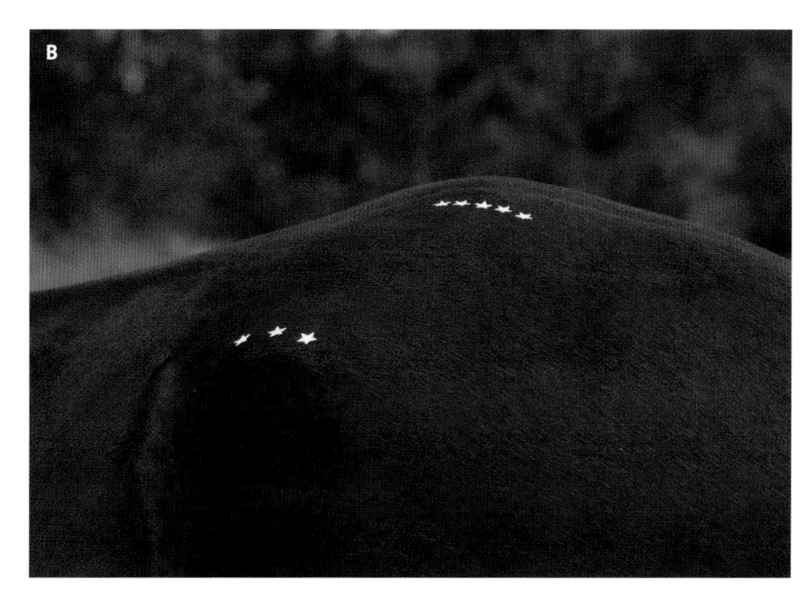

23.2 A & B **Photo A shows a horse with an easily seen tuber coxae and "peak" of the rear end. The line of five stars in B indicates where you place your right hand when working on the horse's left side—along the sacrum, just to the rear of the peak of the rear end (see also fig. 22.3, p. 132)—and the line of three stars shows where your left hand goes, above the tuber coxae.**

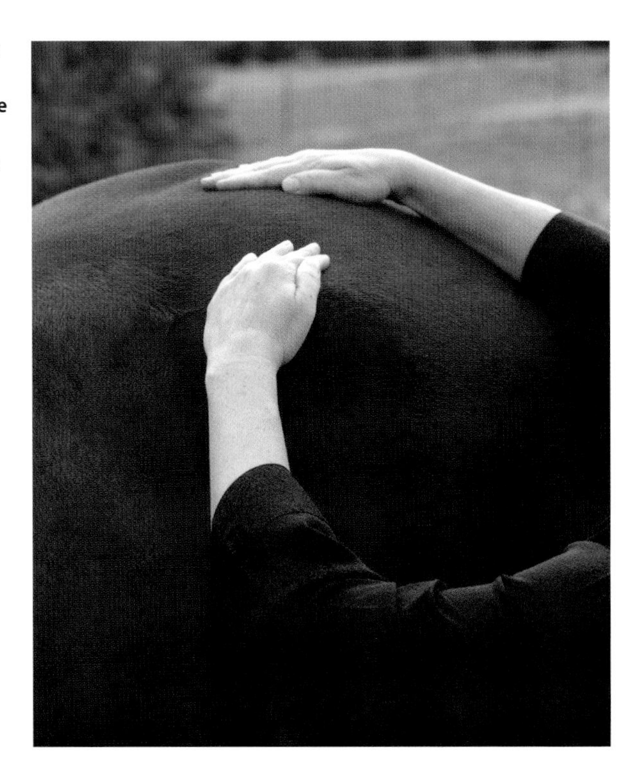

23.3 When doing this Checkup on the left side of the horse, my left hand gently pulls down while the right hand feels for movement.

Checkup Directions

FUNCTION: The sacroiliac joints are extremely important. All the force from the hind limbs travels through them in order to propel the horse forward.

RANGE OF MOTION: The sacroiliac joints' range of motion is much larger than you can check while the horse is in a standing position. The range of motion that you do check is via the tuber coxae (point of the hip). The tuber coxae can move one-half to 1 inch vertically.

While moving the tuber coxae, you also feel the sacroiliac joint movement, which is underneath 4 to 6 inches of muscle. Consequently, it takes practice to feel the sacroiliac motion.

HOW TO

Stand at the horse's hip with the horse standing square. Place one hand along the near side of the sacrum and the other on top of the tuber coxae (figs. 23.2 A & B).

Gently pull down vertically on the tuber coxae. Ideally, the point of hip should move down one-half to 1 inch (fig. 23.3). Meanwhile, feel the movement under your hand next to the sacrum as the tuber coxae moves up and down: You are feeling the movement of the sacroiliac joint.

As you practice, you'll get a feel for the quality of this motion. For now, just be sure that you feel the same amount of movement on both sides of the horse. More movement is better than less, but they need to be equal on both sides.

Diagnosis

If the tuber coxae doesn't move at all, the sacroiliac joint is definitely subluxated. If one side has a different amount, or quality, of movement than the other side, you most likely have a chiropractic subluxation in the sacroiliac joint(s).

Summary: SACROILIAC JOINT

- When evidence of subluxation, call chiropractor.
- When Checkup is fine but common symptoms remain, check for:
    - Subluxations at: sacrum; intertransverse joint; hocks; stifle (pp. 130, 126, 145, 141)
    - Hock or stifle issues such as OCD (osteochondritis dessicans) arthritis or lax stifle ligaments
    - Vitamin and/or mineral deficiency

BODY CHECKUP

THE HIP JOINT 24

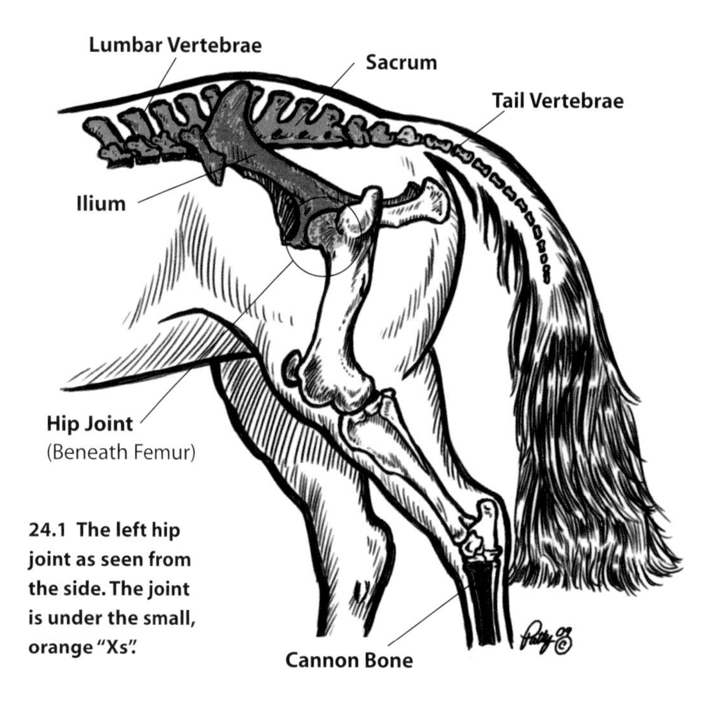

24.1 The left hip joint as seen from the side. The joint is under the small, orange "Xs".

I was once called to help Allie, a lovely, gentle Percheron mare. Although only five years old, she was destined to be a broodmare because she had run into a tree as a youngster and had a "dropped hip." (This refers to the end part of the tuber coxae—point of the hip—being hit with enough force to literally "drop it down" 1 to 2 inches.) Her owners were having difficulty getting her bred.

Nerves to the uterus and ovaries come from the pelvic area. It's common to see chiropractic subluxations of the lumbar, sacrum, and sacroiliac be a cause of ovulation, breeding, and pregnancy difficulties. As I checked Allie (from a very large stepstool) I found that her main problems were in her hind-end area. Her sacrum, sacroiliac, lumbar, and right hip were subluxated. All of these subluxations were most likely caused by the "dropped hip." The muscles attached to the dropped hip "relocate" along with it, causing continuous difficulties in musculoskeletal alignment.

Once Allie was adjusted, she "took" (was confirmed bred) on her next heat cycle. We maintained her chiropractic adjustments every two to three months through the pregnancy until one month before her due date. (It is unwise to adjust pregnant animals—or people—in the last 30 days of pregnancy.) Allie delivered a healthy filly right on time.

HIP JOINT CHALLENGE LEVEL ☆☆☆
Locating Anatomic Area: ☆☆☆
Positioning of Horse or Handler: ☆☆☆
Subtle Range of Motion: ☆☆☆
Complex Evaluation of Checkup: ☆☆☆

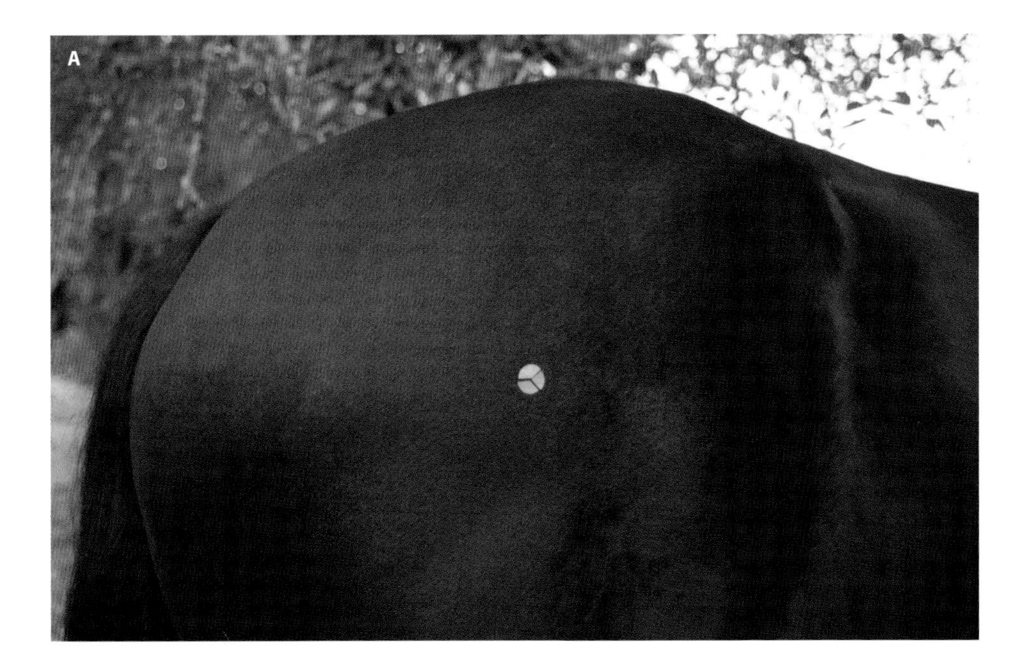

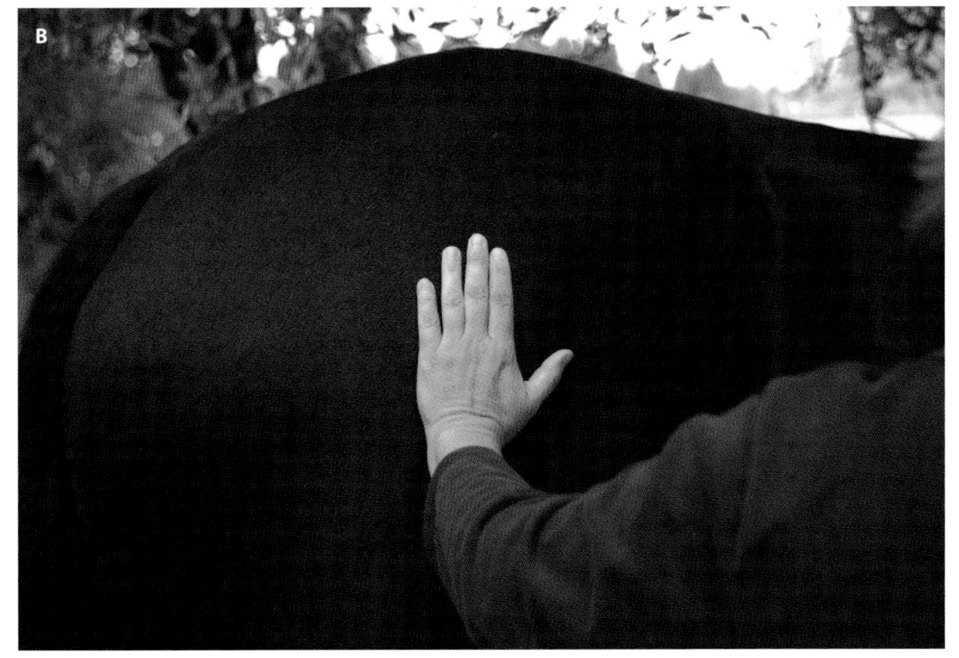

24.2 A & B The green dot in A indicates the hip joint, and B shows the correct hand placement over the hip joint for the Checkup.

What I Mean By "Hip"

When I refer to the hip, I'm talking about the anatomic hip joint. Many people refer to the horse's hip as the entire hind-end gluteal area (or rump), but in this book, hip always means hip joint.

Common Symptoms

BEHAVIORAL OR PERFORMANCE SYMPTOMS

Very Common

- Walking stiffly in the hind end

Frequent

- Short-striding in the hind end
- Struggles with hind-end lateral work

Occasional

- Not "tracking up" (the hind feet not landing straight in the prints left by the front feet)
- When standing, one hind leg turns out to the side

PHYSICAL SYMPTOMS: CURRENT OR PRIOR

- Stocking up in hind legs
- Hip or gluteal muscles have tight bands or knots
- Low-heel/high-heel syndrome in the hind feet, chronic

- Hock or stifle problems
- Sacral or sacroiliac subluxations

Checkup Directions

FUNCTION: The hip joint of the horse is a ball-and-socket joint similar to our own. The hip transfers the forward propulsive power from the hind legs to the pelvis.

RANGE OF MOTION: Stand up on one leg and move your other leg around in a circle about 2 to 4 inches off the floor, and you'll get the idea of the hip joint's range of motion that you are evaluating.

HOW TO

This Checkup is for the actual hip joint, not any other part of the rear end. It can best be felt in the center of the horse's hind-end region (figs. 24.2 A & B). (NOTE: If you are not certain you are on the hip joint, simply continue with the Checkup steps below, but move your hand around the area until you find the spot with the most movement.)

Stand next to the horse's hind leg and hold it by the cannon bone with one hand just off the ground, approximately 2 to 4 inches. Place the palm of your free hand over the hip joint to evaluate the hip joint's movement. Keeping the horse's foot as level

24.3 A–C When checking the hip joint, move the horse's hind leg in a complete circle while feeling the hip with the other hand to see if it is functioning properly.

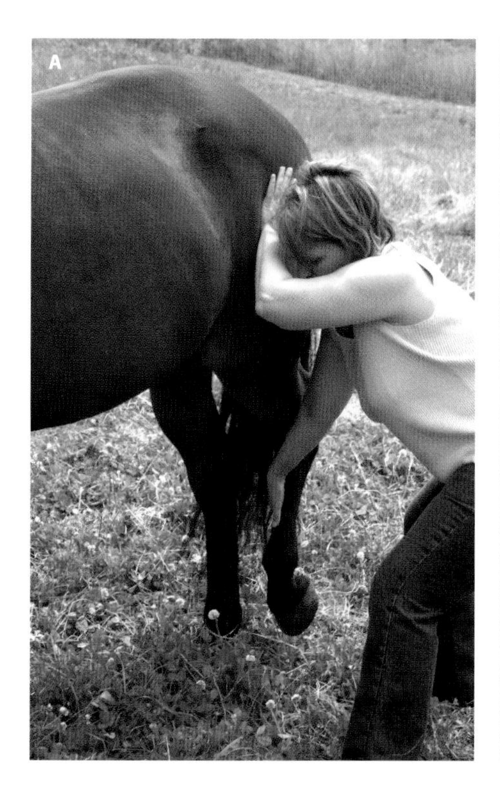

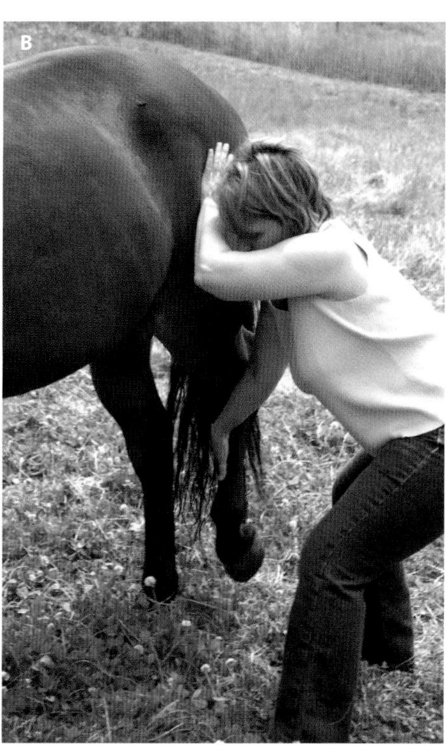

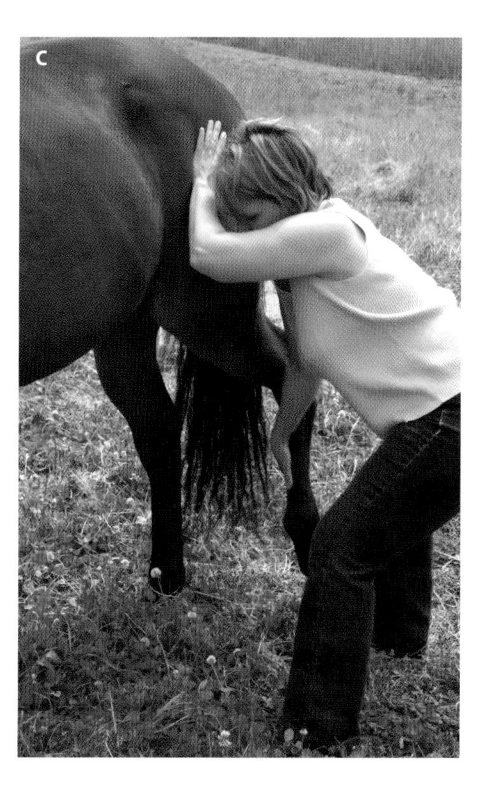

to the ground as possible, move the leg in a full circle, both clockwise and counterclockwise (figs. 24.3 A–C). The circle's diameter should be approximately 12 inches, though a few inches smaller or larger is fine.

Diagnosis

Because many horses overuse their hip muscles to compensate for subluxations and/or hock problems, hip muscles can be tight and sore. This makes this a complicated Checkup to evaluate. I recommend evaluating the hip in two ways. First, the foot should be able to travel through the circular path in both directions without stopping, "sticking," or moving off the path. When it does so consistently each time you get to one section of the circle, the hip joint is subluxated.

Second, feel the movement of the hip joint itself, via the muscles, under your palm over the hip joint. This is a more subtle feeling and takes practice. Hip muscles suddenly tensing up as the foot travels the circle may indicate hip subluxation.

Summary: HIP JOINT

- When leg does not go around circle cleanly and hip muscles tighten up, hip is likely subluxated, call chiropractor.
    - When hip muscles tighten up regardless of foot's ability to go around circle, first check if muscles are sore when gently massaged with the foot on the ground. If yes, resolve sore muscles first, call massage therapist and/or veterinarian.
    - When foot can go around circle and the muscles do not tighten up: Hooray! The hip is fine.

- When no subluxations but still see symptoms of a hip joint problem, check for:
    - Subluxations at: sacroiliac; sacrum; intertransverse joint; lumbar vertebrae—especially L6 (pp. 134, 130, 126, 122)
    - Hock issues
    - Stifle issues
    - Hoof-wall imbalance
    - Hind-foot angles incorrect and/or uneven
    - Vitamin and/or mineral deficiency

BODY CHECKUP 25
THE STIFLE

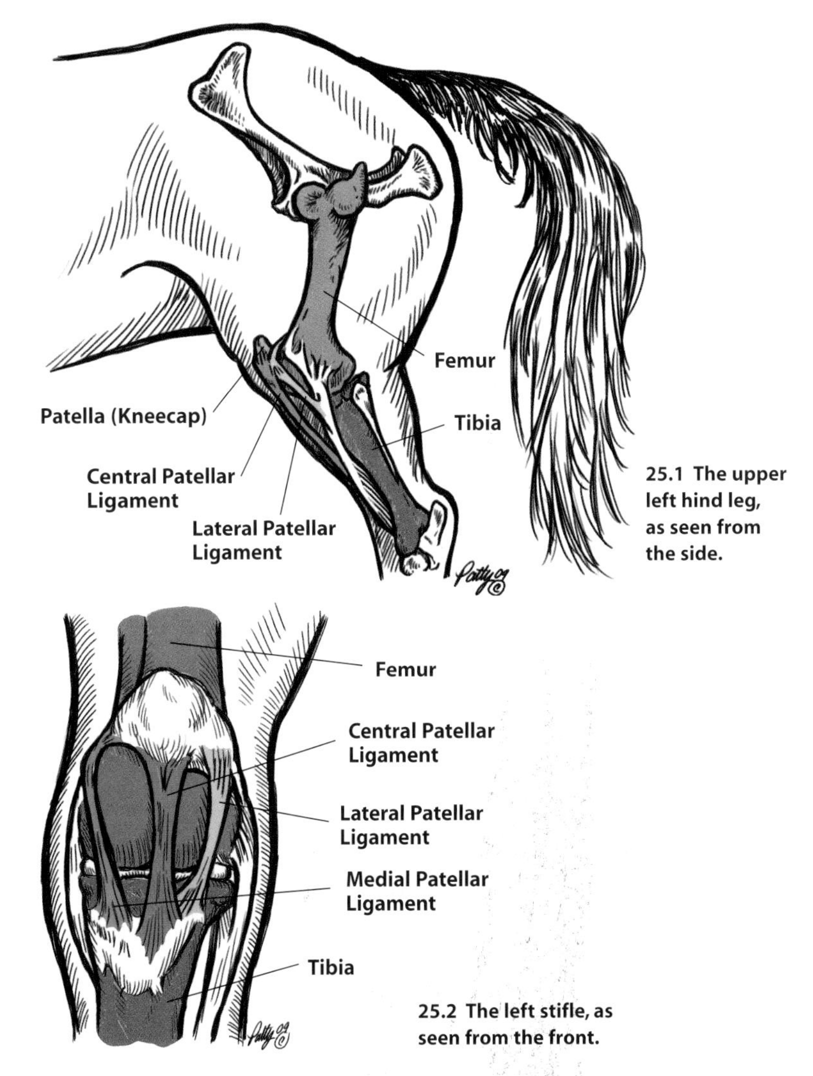

25.1 The upper left hind leg, as seen from the side.

25.2 The left stifle, as seen from the front.

"Well, my horse has a locking stifle, and I'm just wondering if you can do anything about it?" This loud query came from a short older gentleman in a red-plaid flannel shirt, tan hat, and amazingly old cowboy boots. I had just met Dan and his prize Azteca stallion, Joe.

Dan continued, "I've had three vets look at him and no one can fix him. They just keep on talkin' and talkin' and no one fixes him. He's only four years old and he is a star at mounted shooting! I want him FIXED."

I paused and waited before replying because I wanted to know if he was going to spit some chew my way. None came. "Can you walk him a bit for me so I can see what he's doing?" I asked.

"I'm not an invalid, you know," He replied. "I can walk him just fine. It's Joe that can't walk. And nobody can FIX him." And he walked him off down the barn aisle.

Joe walked with a funny gait. His left hind took a normal step forward, but in mid-stride the foot would

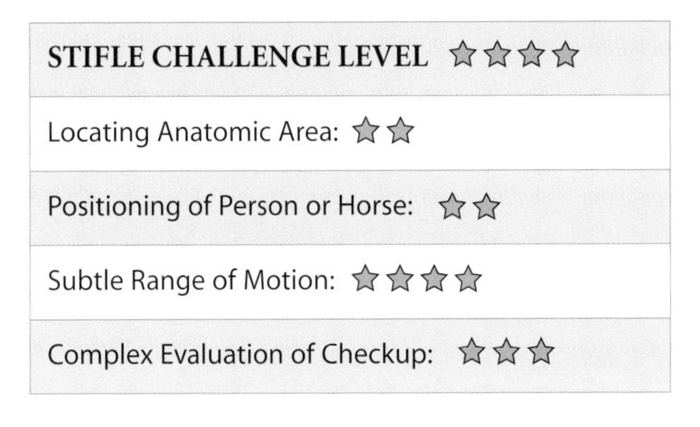

STIFLE CHALLENGE LEVEL ☆☆☆☆
Locating Anatomic Area: ☆☆
Positioning of Person or Horse: ☆☆
Subtle Range of Motion: ☆☆☆☆
Complex Evaluation of Checkup: ☆☆☆

slam down to the ground. His stifle never did lock. I expect Dan used the term generically.

"When the other vets were talking, did they mention fibrotic myopathy?" I asked.

"Well, they just kept talkin' and talkin' and nobody FIXED him!" Dan replied, then after a pause, "Well, I guess they might of mentioned something like that, but nobody FIXED him."

"Sir," I said, "I am going to give 'fixing Joe' my best shot. He has fibrotic myopathy, but with chiropractic and acupuncture we can definitely improve his gait."

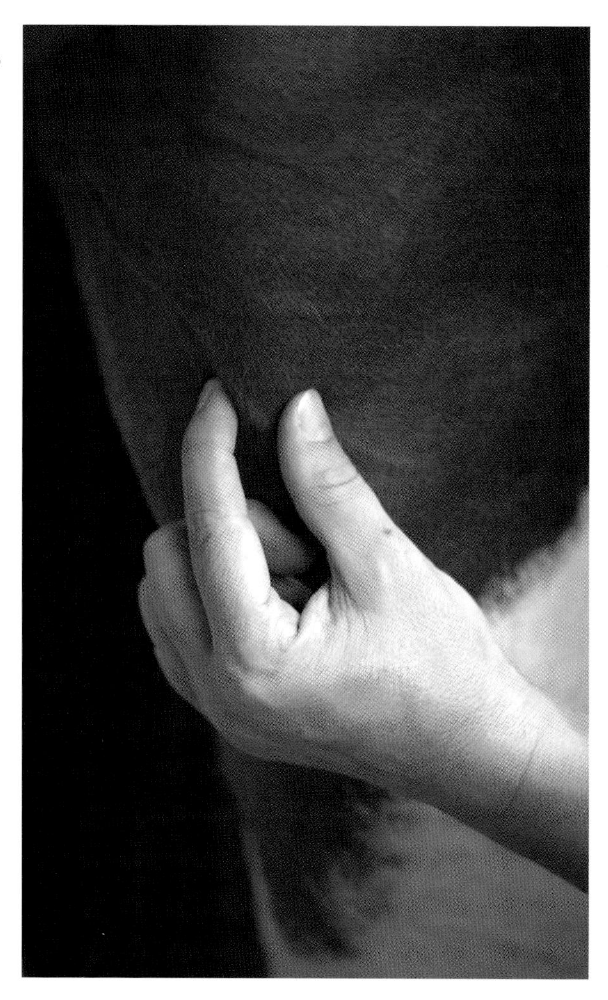

25.3 I demonstrate feeling the tension in the central patellar ligament.

Fibrotic myopathy is a tightening of the hamstring due to calcification. It is usually caused by trauma. It keeps the leg muscle from being able to stretch enough to step forward with a full stride. Chiropractic and acupuncture treatments definitely can improve horses with this problem. In my experience, there is always at least a 50-percent improvement and sometimes more than that.

Common Symptoms

BEHAVIORAL OR PERFORMANCE SYMPTOMS

Very Common

- Stiff in hind end
- Struggles with hind-end lateral work

Frequent

- Reluctance to make tight turns
- Difficulty with collection or impulsion

Occasional

- Short-striding behind
- Standing with the hind leg turned out to the side
- Reluctance to jump
- Goes wide on turns
- Reluctance to go downhill
- Prefers to trot over other gaits
- "Phantom" lameness behind
- Hind end has uneven takeoff when jumping

PHYSICAL SYMPTOMS: CURRENT OR PRIOR

- Hock issues, particularly in the opposite hind leg
- Stifle issues or injury
- Lumbar subluxations, recurrent

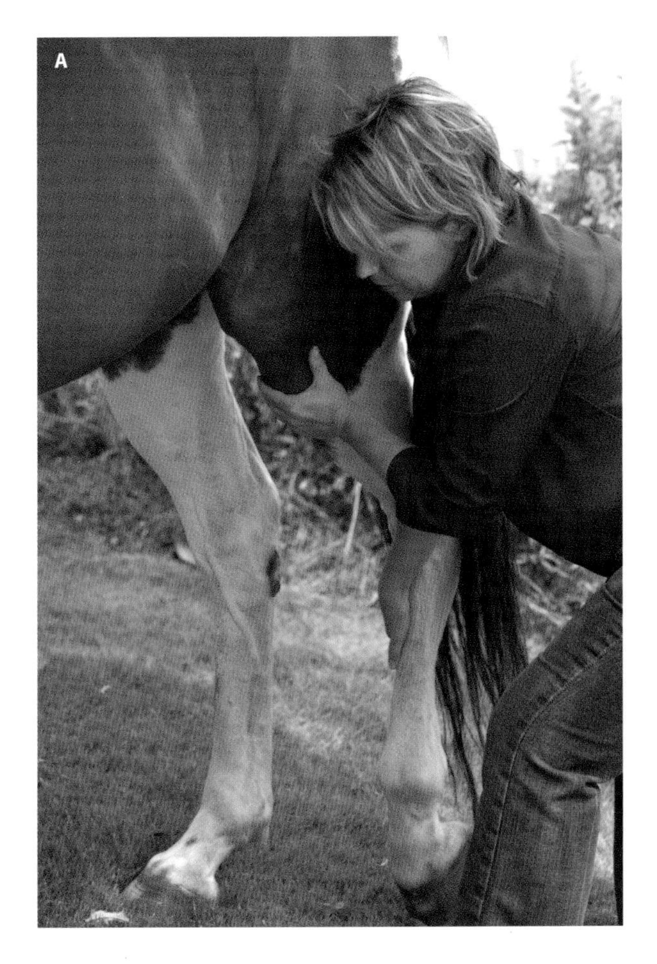

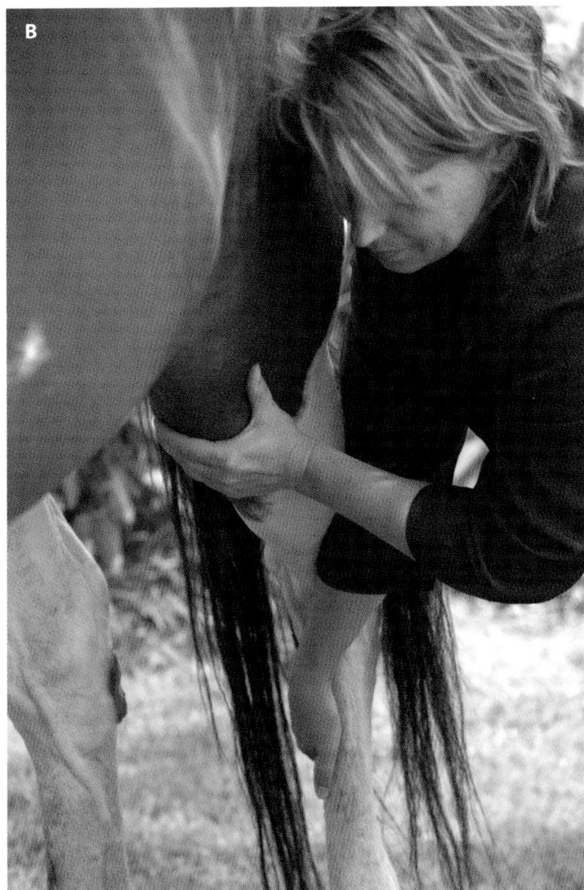

25.4 A & B
During the stifle Checkup, notice that the horse lightly rests his left hind leg in the "toe-touch" position.

Checkup Directions

FUNCTION: The stifle joint is analogous to our knee. The stifle's function is primarily that of assisting forward propulsion.

RANGE OF MOTION: The stifle flexes and extends just like our knee. It also has a very small side-to-side movement, less than one-quarter inch.

HOW TO

TEST 1

One part of this examination is to check the ligament tension in the stifle. The three major ligaments of the knee are the lateral, central, and medial patellar ligaments. These are shown in the anatomic illustrations on p. 141. Simply feel the ligaments for equal tension, both on the leg when it is standing and when it is resting (fig. 25.3). Feel the ligaments by pushing down as you bring your fingers across them (that is, from side to side) rather than along them. Push down with the same amount of force that you would use to comfortably massage your own ligaments on the inside of your wrist.

TEST 2

The second part of the exam involves having the horse "rest" his leg again, ideally just "toe-touching" the ground while the remainder of the leg is relaxed. When the horse is uncomfortable or doesn't understand the request, have a second person hold the leg just off the ground. Alternatively, if you're feeling particularly agile, you can hold the horse's leg off the ground using your own leg.

Once the leg is positioned in a relaxed manner, hold the cannon bone still with one hand while moving the lower part of the stifle (tibia) side to side with the other (figs. 25.4 A & B).

Diagnosis

TEST 1: If you notice that one ligament is too loose or too tight as compared to the other two, especially on the resting leg, you most likely have a stifle subluxation.

TEST 2: You should feel even movement on both sides of the stifle, without signs of tension or discomfort. This movement is very small, approximately one-quarter inch. It will often feel like more of a "give" than true "motion." When there is no movement to one side (this feels like trying to push against solid rock), you most likely have a subluxated stifle. Another possibility is potentially stifle arthritis, which is best detected with a traditional veterinary flexion exam and X-rays.

Summary: STIFLE

- ▶ When stifle ligaments do not have equal tension or there is uneven movement of the stifle side to side, you may have a subluxation—call chiropractor.
- ▶ When no subluxation suspected, yet symptoms remain, check for:
  - Subluxations at: hock; lumbar vertebrae; sacrum (pp. 145, 122, 130)
  - Stifle arthritis or OCD (osteochondritis dissecans)
  - Hoof-wall imbalance
  - Hind foot angles incorrect and/or uneven

BODY CHECKUP 26 THE HOCK

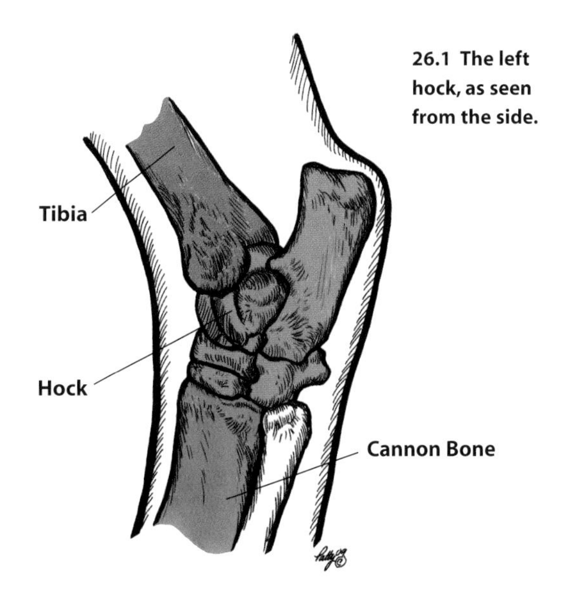

26.1 The left hock, as seen from the side.

You should regularly check for "hock wobble." This is just what it sounds like. Watch your horse walk or trot while standing behind him to see if a hock (one or both) literally wobbles back and forth (right and left) a few times with each footfall.

This can be normal and is not a concern with growing horses, particularly if it is symmetrical on both legs. However, when asymmetrical, or seen in a mature horse, hock wobble is a sign of incorrect alignment. It may be a misalignment at the hock, or anywhere in the hind end. Notice I refer to this as a "misalignment" and not necessarily as a subluxation. Hock wobble may be caused from subluxations, but also can be from other issues such as: incorrect hoof-wall balance, arthritis, muscle damage, or even OCD (osteochondritis dissecans).

Remember, growing horses can be out of alignment and have hock wobble for different periods of time as they go through growth spurts. Just keep checking and make sure it goes away. NOTE: Hock wobble may be normal in gaited horses.

HOCK CHALLENGE LEVEL ☆☆☆
Locating Anatomic Area: ☆
Positioning of Person or Horse: ☆☆
Subtle Range of Motion: ☆☆☆
Complex Evaluation of Checkup: ☆☆☆

Common Symptoms

BEHAVIORAL OR PERFORMANCE SYMPTOMS

Very Common

- Short-striding behind
- Difficulty with collection or impulsion
- Stiff in hind end

Frequent

- Difficulty with gait transitions
- Difficulty with hind-end lateral work

Occasional

- Goes wide on turns

- Difficulty with turns
- "Phantom" lameness in hind end
- Prefers to trot over other gaits
- Uneven hind-end takeoff over jumps

PHYSICAL SYMPTOMS: CURRENT OR PRIOR

- Opposing front leg, history of issues
- Hind foot, incorrect angles
- Hock injury, history of
- Stifle issues on opposing rear leg, chronic
- Sacroiliac or sacrum subluxations, chronic
- Hock or stifle soreness, or other physical problems
- Lumbar subluxations, chronic

Checkup Directions

FUNCTION: The hock is primarily responsible for flexion and extension of the horse's hind leg.

RANGE OF MOTION: The hock has a similar design to the human ankle. Flexing and extending your own ankle will give you an idea of the hock range of motion. Note that human ankles can rotate and bend side to side to a greater extent than the horse's hock.

The hock should be able to flex so that the cannon bone just about touches the femur—the position for the traditional veterinary "hock-flexion" test. While that test gives you good information, it is not the range of motion you will check here. You are looking for the side-to-side motion of the hock by

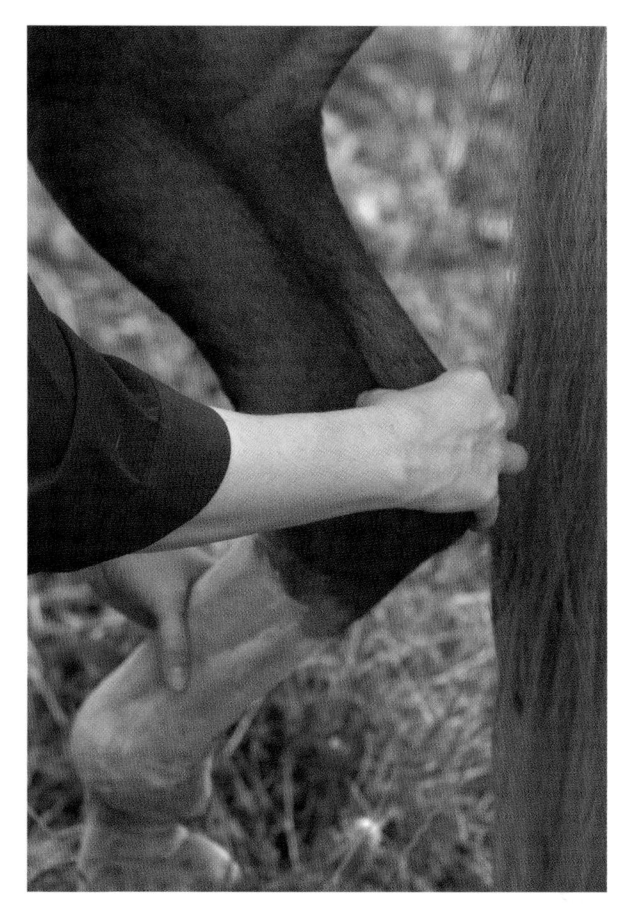

26.2 The correct hand positions for this Checkup: One hand on the mid-cannon bone and the other above the hock.

Where's the Root of the Problem?

The part of the horse's body that is "screaming"—the painful part—is very often not the part with the primary problem. For example, let's say your horse is lame in the left hind leg and a hock flexion test comes back "4 out of 5" (translation: not good). So the horse is in pain from the left hock, and the horse gets much better after a left hock injection. It is possible, in this scenario, that the right sacroiliac joint (p. 134) is so subluxated that it is nonfunctioning, and the left hock has been "picking up the slack," compensating for this. If this is the case, and the right sacroiliac joint problem isn't addressed, then the left hock will continue to need frequent injections.

Keep in mind that recurring problems very often have a different cause than we think they do.

moving the entire leg. Here's why: If you've ever injured a part of your ankle, you may recall that you can "freeze" your ankle in a nonpainful position with your muscles and still walk. However, when you tried to flex it side to side, it is painful. Many horses with hock issues simply "freeze" the hock and continue to use it within a smaller-than-normal range of motion. They use their stifle and hip to compensate and still maintain correct stride length. But when you ask them to "wiggle" their hocks side to side and there's discomfort, you'll get a response.

You are not looking for a pain response such as a muscle flinch with this Checkup, but simply the "freeze." When abnormalities are present, the horse will not allow the hock to be moved from side to side, but will hold it in the neutral position instead.

HOW TO

Hold the leg in a relaxed manner off the ground. On the left side, use your left hand to hold the mid-cannon bone area, while your right hand lightly holds above the hock (fig. 26.2). Take care not to squeeze the gastrocnemius tendon. It's the big tendon just above the point of the hock (fig. 26.3).

Pull with your right hand while pushing with your left, then pull left while pushing right, and repeat. Do these push-pulls quickly and lightly to create a side-to-side "wiggle" through the hock (figs. 26.4 A–C).

Diagnosis

The cannon bone should move, at a minimum, 2 to 3 inches side to side through the "wiggle." If the horse "freezes" the hock, not allowing any wiggling, he either has arthritis or a hock subluxation. Often, with

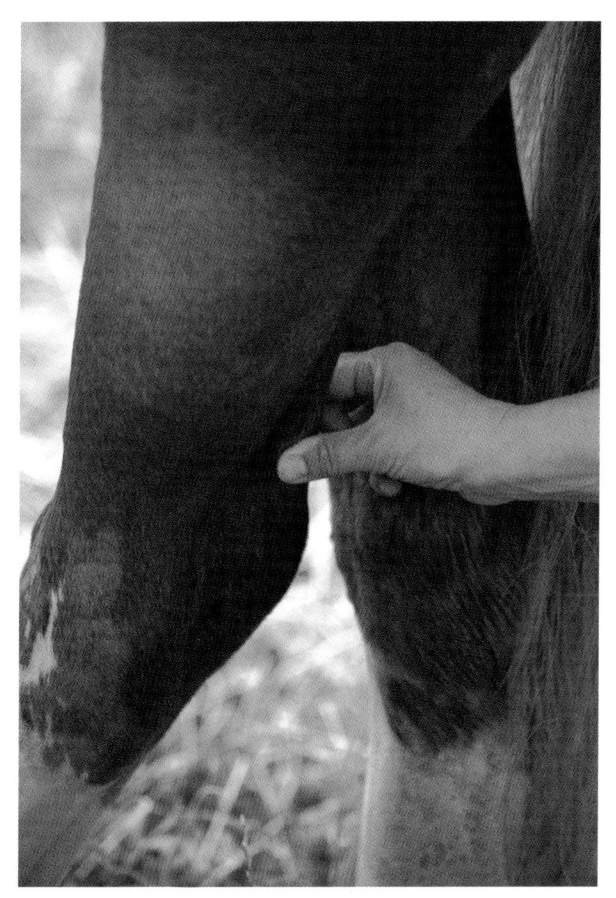

26.3 Here, my thumb and forefinger hold the gastrocnemius tendon, which you must not squeeze during this Checkup.

The Wiggle Exercise

The hock "wiggle" human comparison: Hold up your arm in front of you with your elbow bent about 90 degrees, flop your hand back and forth through its flexion and extension, and you'll see the wiggle through your wrist. If your wrist hurts, you would "freeze" it and not allow the wiggle to happen just as the horse does with a hock subluxation.

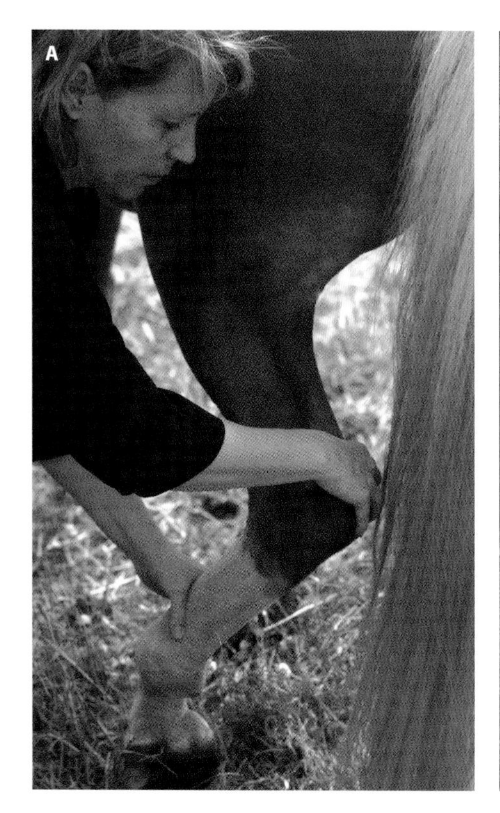

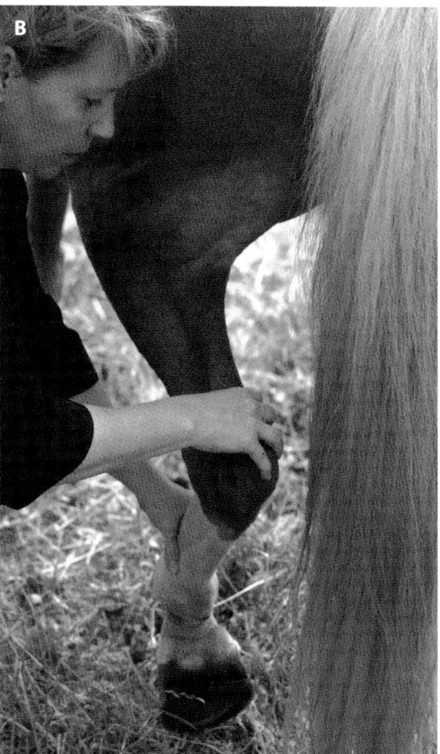

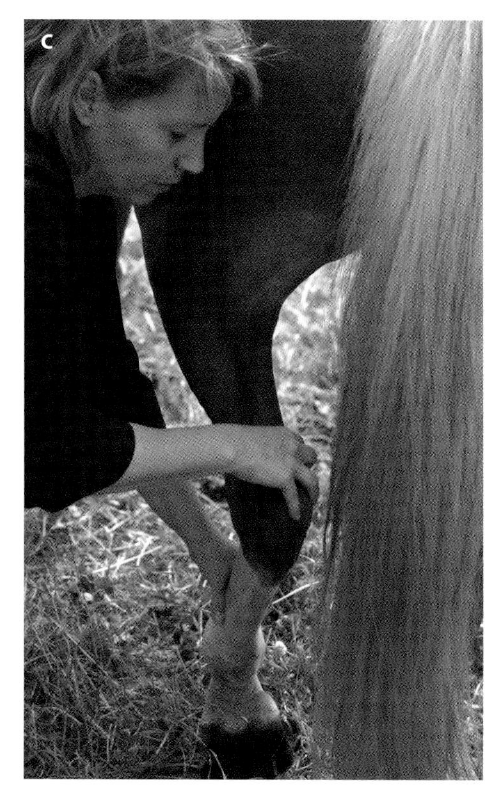

26.4 A–C Note the movement of the hock as I rotate it inward in photo A, to neutral in B, and outward in C.

a subluxated hock, the horse will freeze to one side only. Typically, an arthritic hock freezes in both directions.

Summary: HOCK

- When hock does not "wiggle" evenly to both sides at least 2 to 3 inches, or cannot wiggle to one side at all, call chiropractor.
- When hock is "frozen" in both directions (no "wiggle" whatsoever), call veterinarian.
- When no hock subluxations apparent, but symptoms still exist, check for:
  - Subluxations at: sacrum; sacroiliac joint; lumbar vertebrae; ribs (pp. 130, 134, 122, 117)
  - Stifle issues
  - Vitamin and/or mineral imbalance
  - Saddle fit
  - Hoof-wall imbalance
  - Hind foot angles incorrect and/or uneven

BODY CHECKUP 27 THE TAIL VERTEBRAE

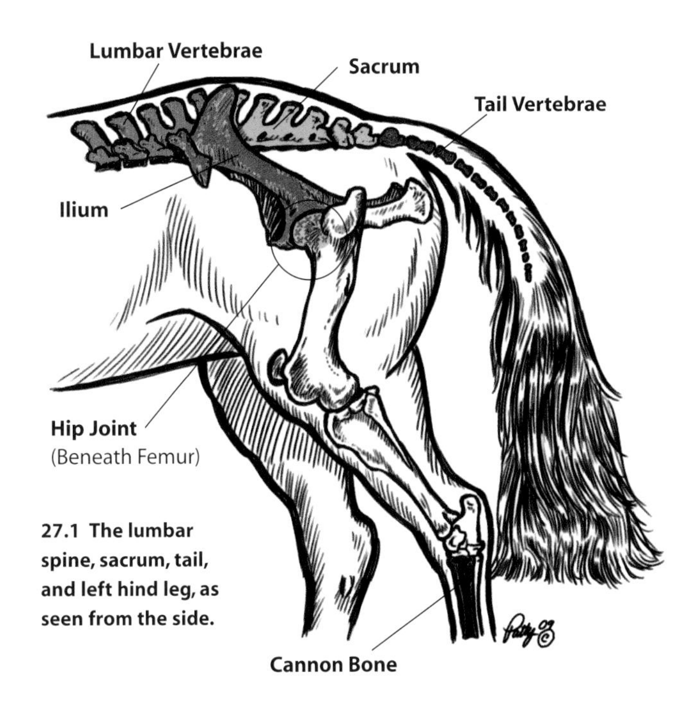

27.1 The lumbar spine, sacrum, tail, and left hind leg, as seen from the side.

A fascinating fact that most people don't realize is that a single subluxated tail vertebra can cause short-striding in the horse's hind end. Here's why: Muscles over the top part of the tail's vertebrae attach to the gluteal (rump) area. There are also muscles on the tail's underside that actually attach to the pelvic floor muscles and are then connected with the abdominal muscles. Consequently, when the tail is subluxated these pelvic floor and abdominal muscles can become overtight—restricting forward movement in the rear legs.

Sometimes when I find a tail subluxation, there is an obvious cause, such as the horse having fallen over

TAIL VERTEBRAE CHALLENGE LEVEL ☆
Locating Anatomic Area: ☆
Positioning of Person or Horse: ☆
Subtle Range of Motion: ☆
Complex Evaluation of Checkup: ☆

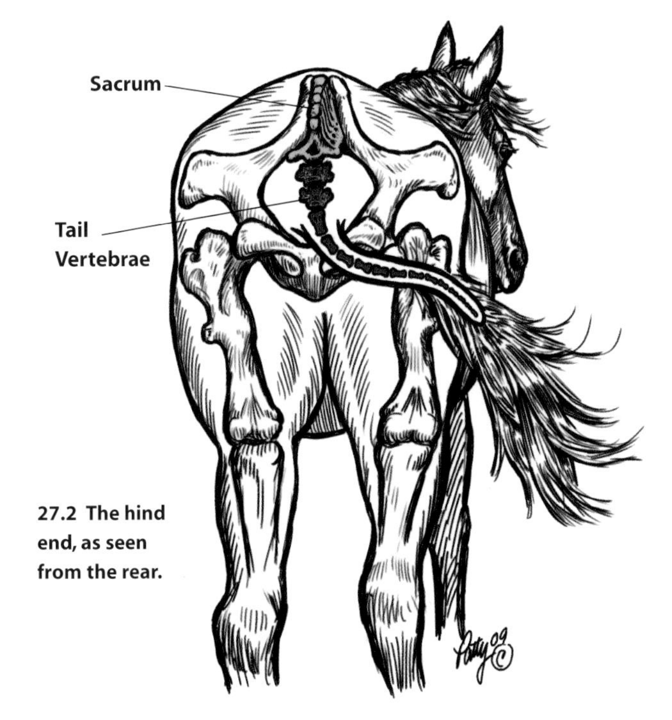

27.2 The hind end, as seen from the rear.

backward in the past, or the current or prior use of a crupper. Other times there is no known reason for the tail subluxation. I have found that with some horses, a tail subluxation can be traced back to the type of handling they had as a foal. Most foals are occasionally held around the chest and by the tail. (NOTE: When you restrain a foal using the tail, be sure to lift the tail straight up vertically. If you pull the tail toward the head, it can cause tail subluxations.)

Common Symptoms

BEHAVIORAL OR PERFORMANCE SYMPTOMS

Very Common

- Tail-clamping when tail is touched

Frequent

- Tail held to one side, when moving or at rest

Occasional

- Difficulty with collection or impulsion
- Difficulty with hind-end lateral work
- "Phantom" lameness in hind end

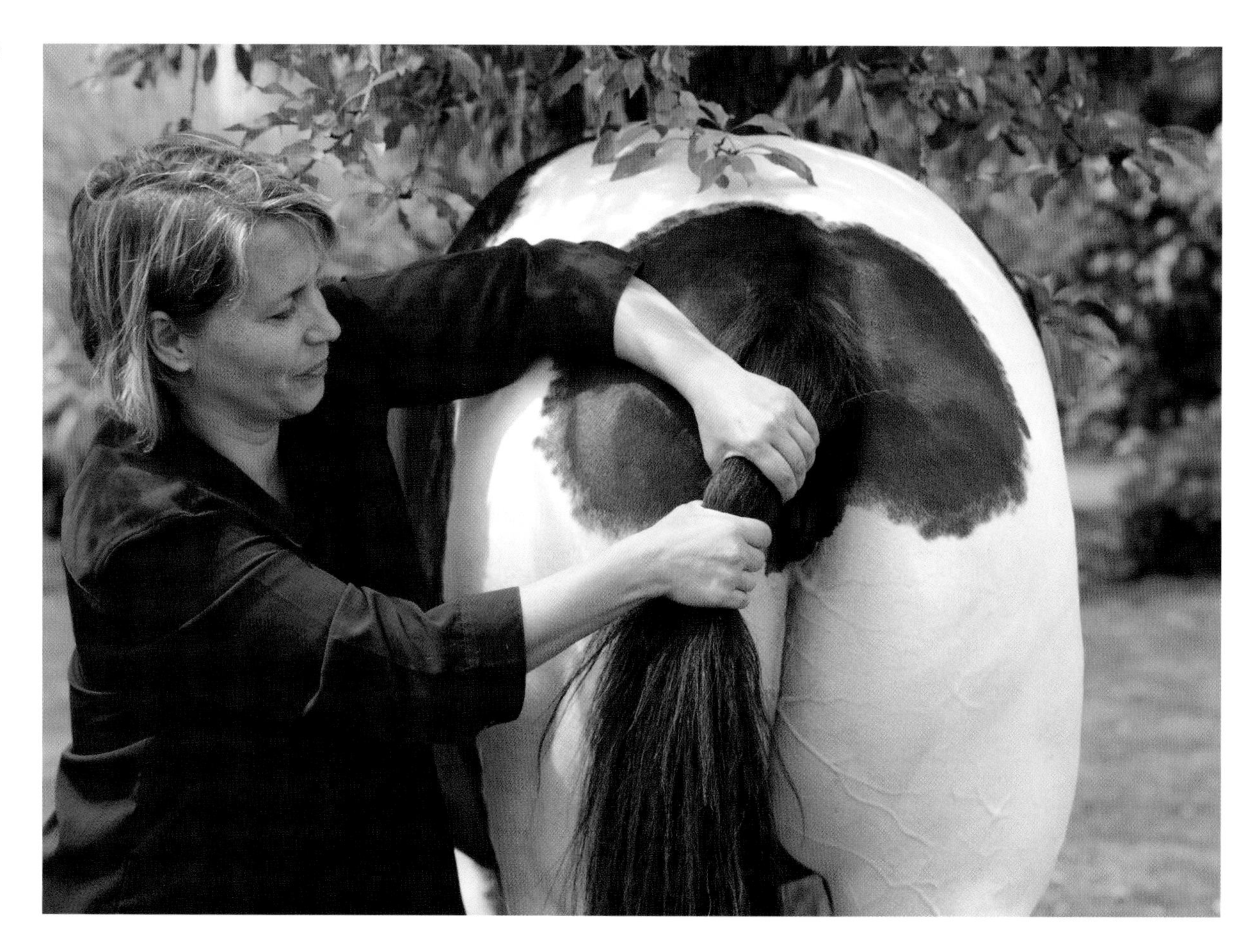

27.3 The correct position for this Checkup, off to one side.

PHYSICAL SYMPTOMS: CURRENT OR PRIOR

- Crupper use, history of
- Tail of foal held too forcefully and/or overflexed
- A fall over backward, incidence of
- Sacral subluxation, history of
- Hind-leg muscles asymmetrical
- Lumbar subluxations, recurrent
- Stocking up in hind end

Checkup Directions

FUNCTION: The tail is used for many balancing functions (as well as a flyswatter). The gluteal (hind-end) muscles attach to the muscles on top of the "tail head," while the pelvic-floor muscles connect to the muscles underneath. When any of the hind-end muscles has an uneven strain on it, the tail is used as a compensation device, often carried to one side.

RANGE OF MOTION: The number of total tail vertebrae ranges from 15 to 21. The first two tail vertebrae compose the "tail head" and are essentially inside the pelvis. That is why we are unable to check the first two tail vertebrae with this Checkup. The remaining tail vertebrae move around in a circular range of motion. The middle tail vertebrae have more movement capability than either the very top or very bottom vertebrae. Tail range of motion varies with breed and the horse's relaxation of the tail. It's important that each individual tail vertebra moves fluidly around its circular pathway.

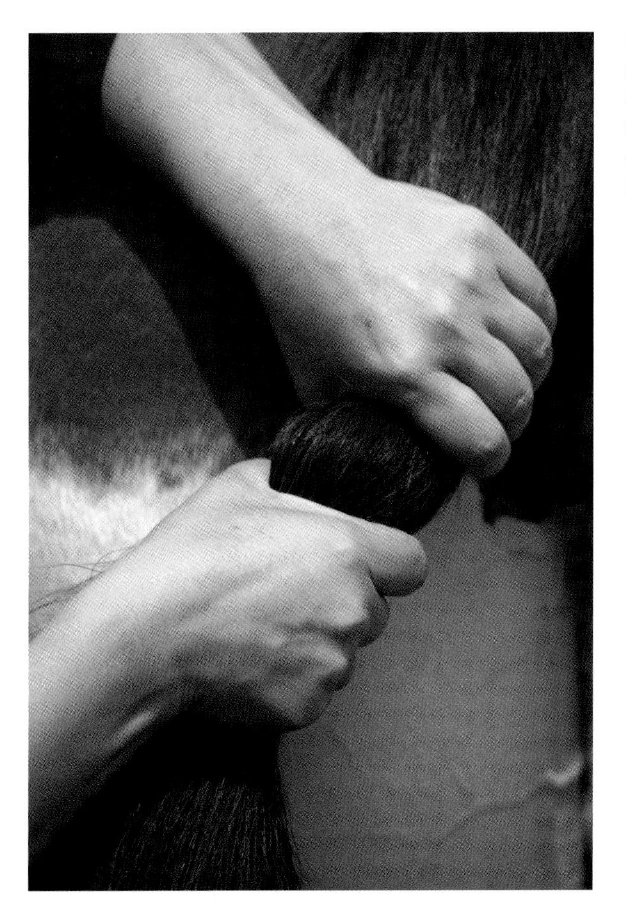

27.4 Each hand, at the top and bottom, holds a tail vertebra, with one vertebra in between.

HOW TO

Always stand to the side of the horse during this exam—not directly behind. Even the most well-mannered animal may kick when his tail hurts (fig. 27.3). Hold the tail head with one hand, "skip" a vertebra, and then hold the following vertebra with your other hand (so one vertebra is "loose" between your two hands—fig. 27.4).

Rotate the bottom tail vertebra around in a circle as you hold the vertebra in your top hand still (fig. 27.5). The tail vertebra in the middle should

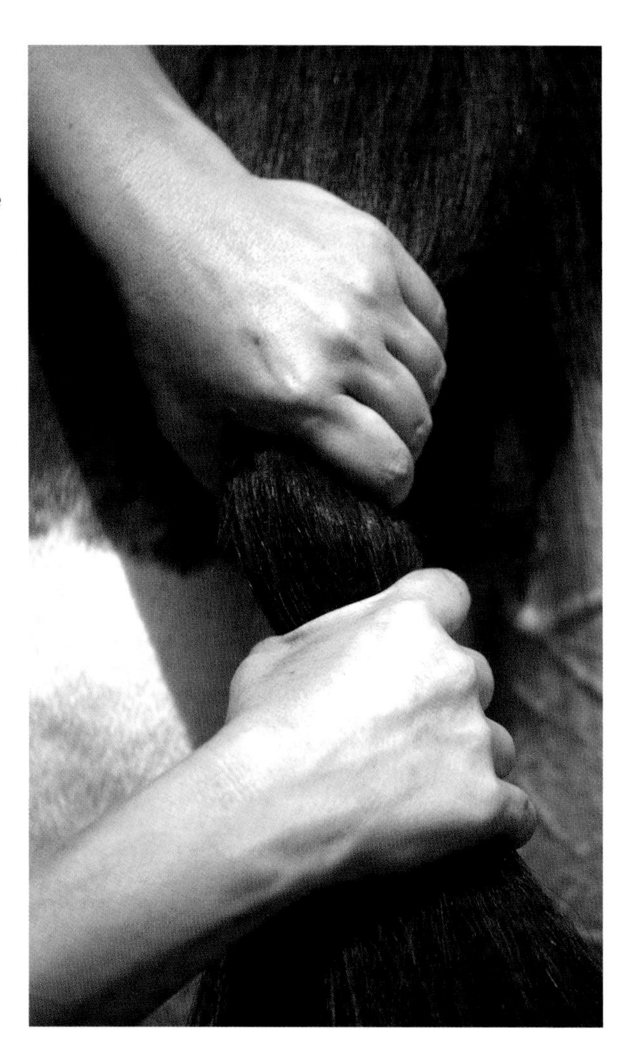

27.5 Rotating the bottom tail vertebra. Note the considerable ability of the tail vertebra to move to the right.

move easily through its circular path. Also do side-to-side and forward and backward movements. Evaluate for equal distance as well as fluidity of movement. There should be no feeling of resistance to the motion.

When you're ready to check the next tail vertebra, slide both your hands down one vertebra and repeat the range of motion evaluation. Continue until you come to the end of the tail.

Diagnosis

Some horses may have broken their tail at some point, but it may not be misshapen at the broken section. A previously broken, though now healed, tail section will not move at all. When it moves in one direction, but not another, it is more likely subluxated than previously broken.

Summary: TAIL VERTEBRAE

- Tail vertebra that does not easily move through a circular path may be subluxated, call chiropractor.
- When the tail Checkup is fine, but symptoms are still apparent, check for subluxations at: sacrum; sacroiliac joint; intertransverse joint; hock joint; stifle (pp. 130, 134, 126, 145, 141)
- Hock or stifle issues

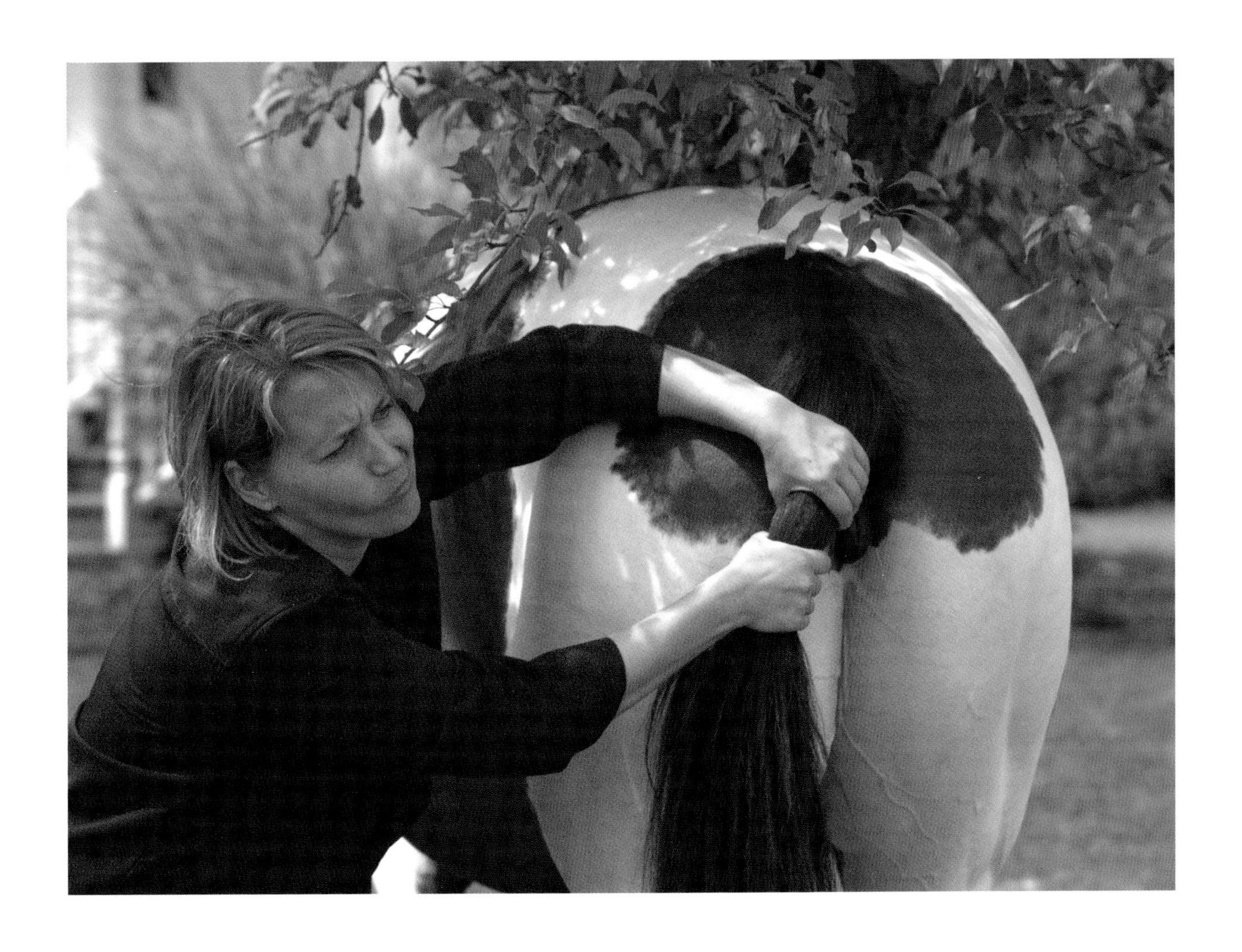

You have just finished the entire program of chiropractic Body Checkups. Congratulations! You can now help your horse remain pain-free and performing well…and hopefully, you do not look like this confused author at the end of the day!

APPENDIX A

Top 10 Complaints List and Problem-Solving Flow Charts

In no particular order the most common issues I've seen during my career as a veterinarian and a chiropractor are listed in the box at right.

Because these issues are so common, I've created quick-reference flow charts to help those dealing with them to formulate a plan of action and follow it. You can find one for each of these complaints on the pages that follow.

TOP 10 COMPLAINTS	
1	Short-striding (or off) in front
2	Short-striding (or off) behind
3	Head-shy or ear-shy
4	Difficulty picking up, maintaining, or changing leads
5	Difficulty with collection or impulsion
6	Difficulty with bending
7	"Girthy"
8	Travels wide and/or drops shoulder on turns
9	Rider feels crooked or saddle slips to one side
10	Horse feels stiff or is cold-backed

1. SHORT-STRIDING (OR OFF) IN FRONT

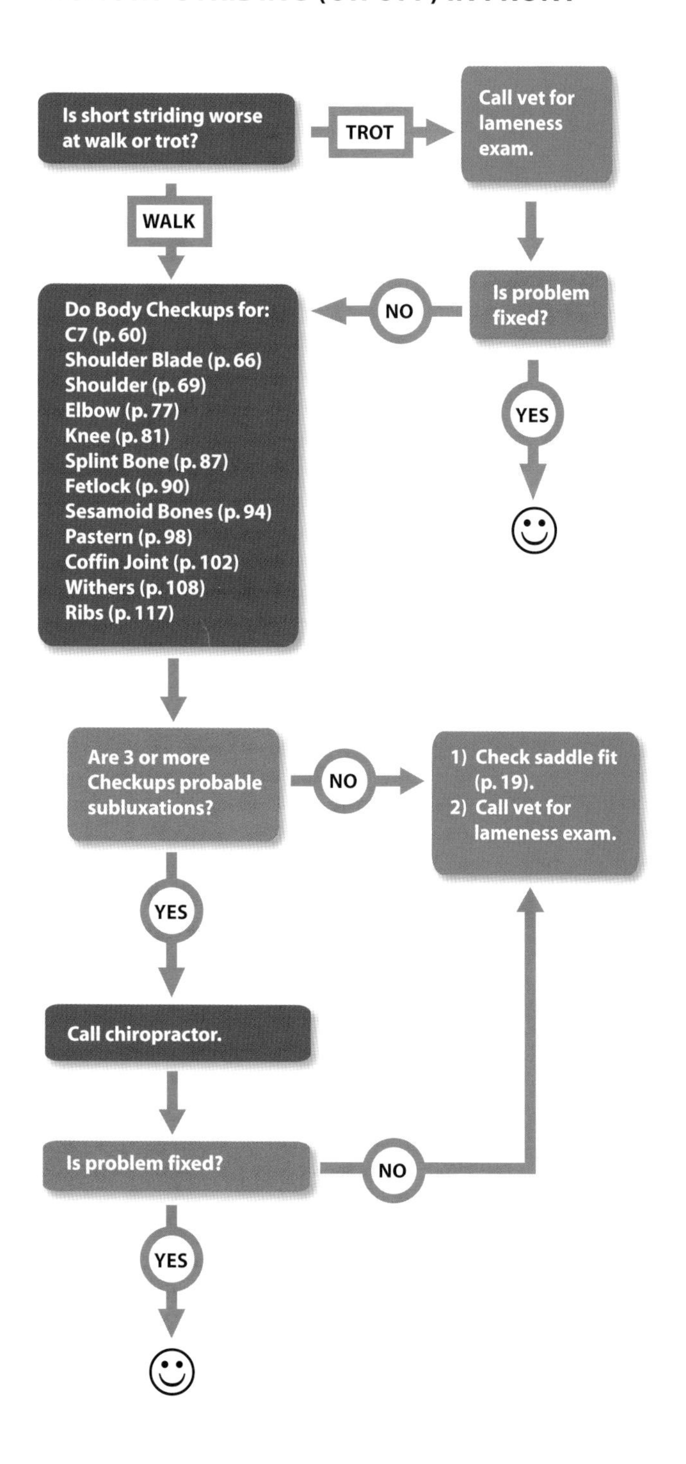

2. SHORT-STRIDING (OR OFF) BEHIND

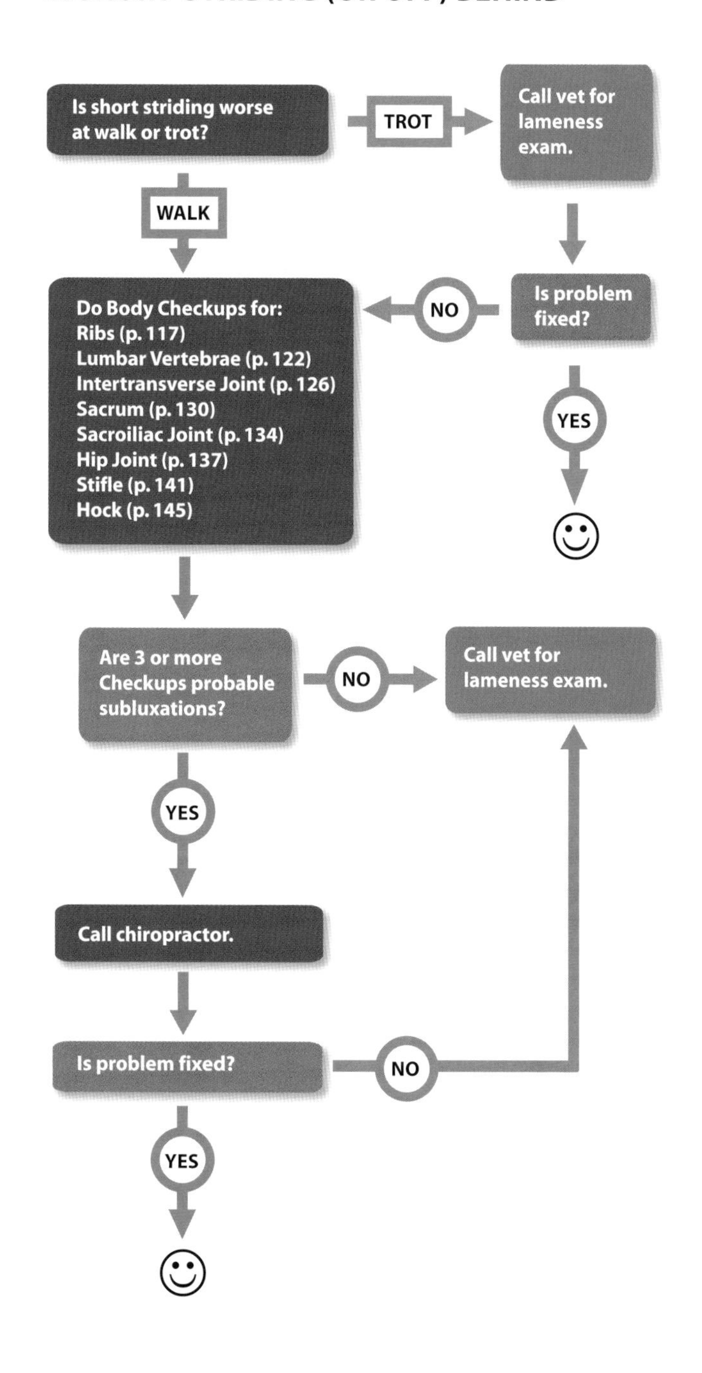

3. HEAD-SHY OR EAR-SHY

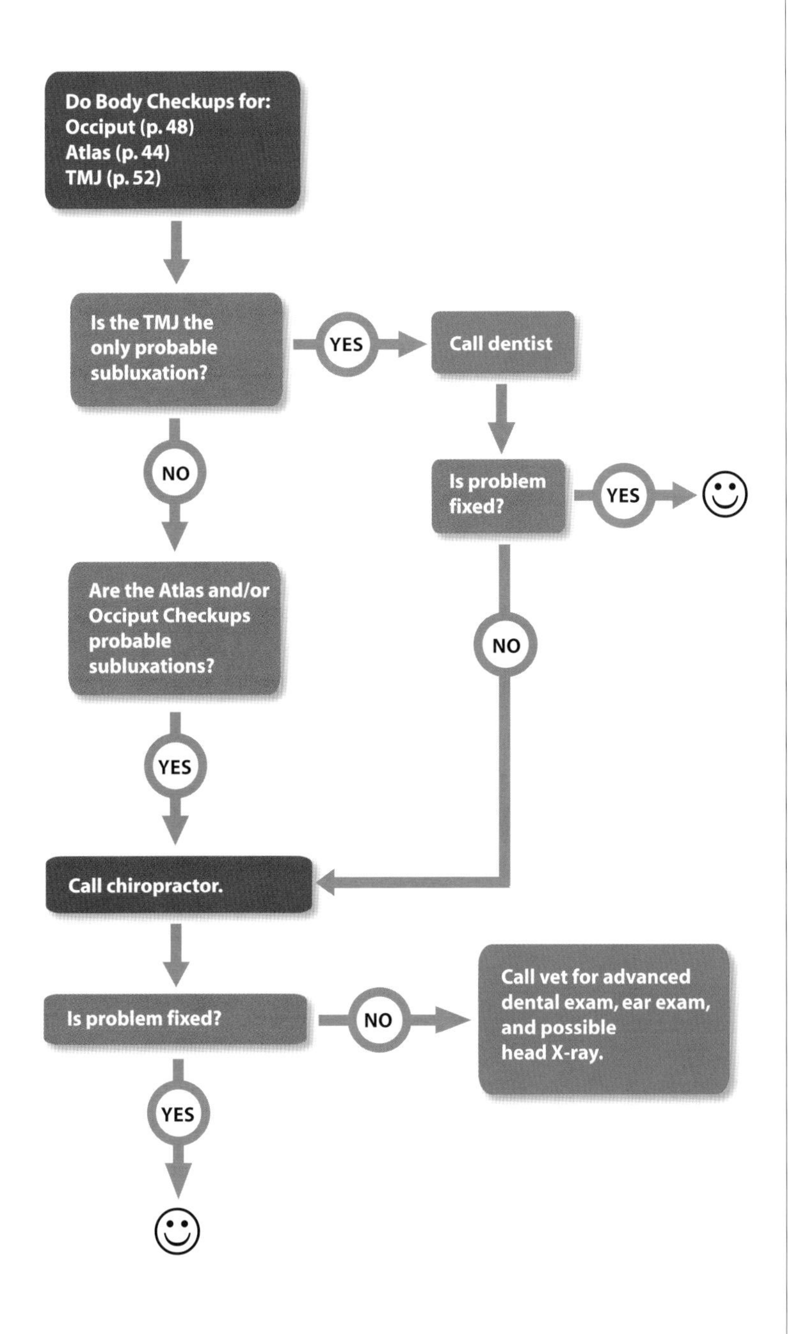

4. DIFFICULTY PICKING UP, MAINTAINING, OR CHANGING LEADS

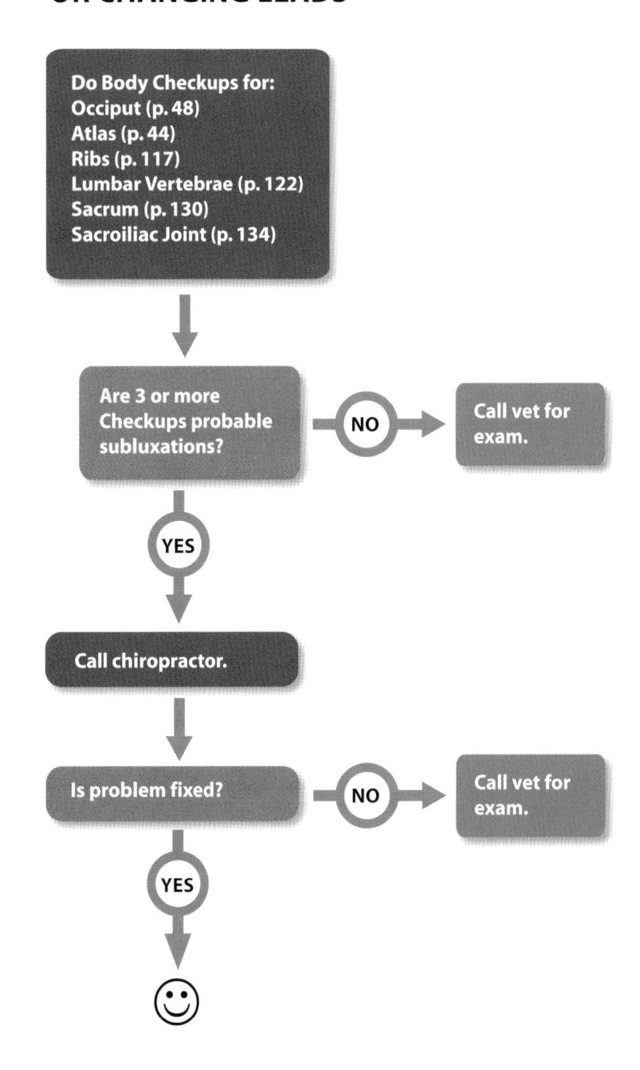

5. DIFFICULTY WITH COLLECTION OR IMPULSION

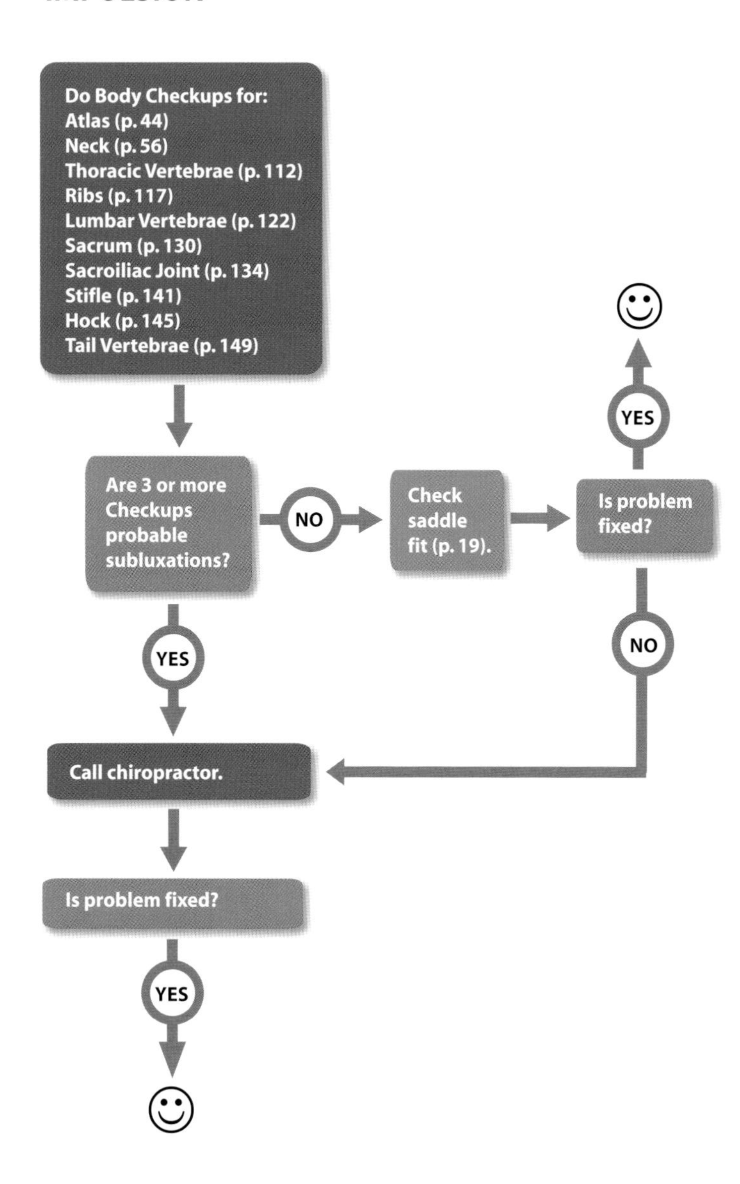

6. DIFFICULTY WITH BENDING

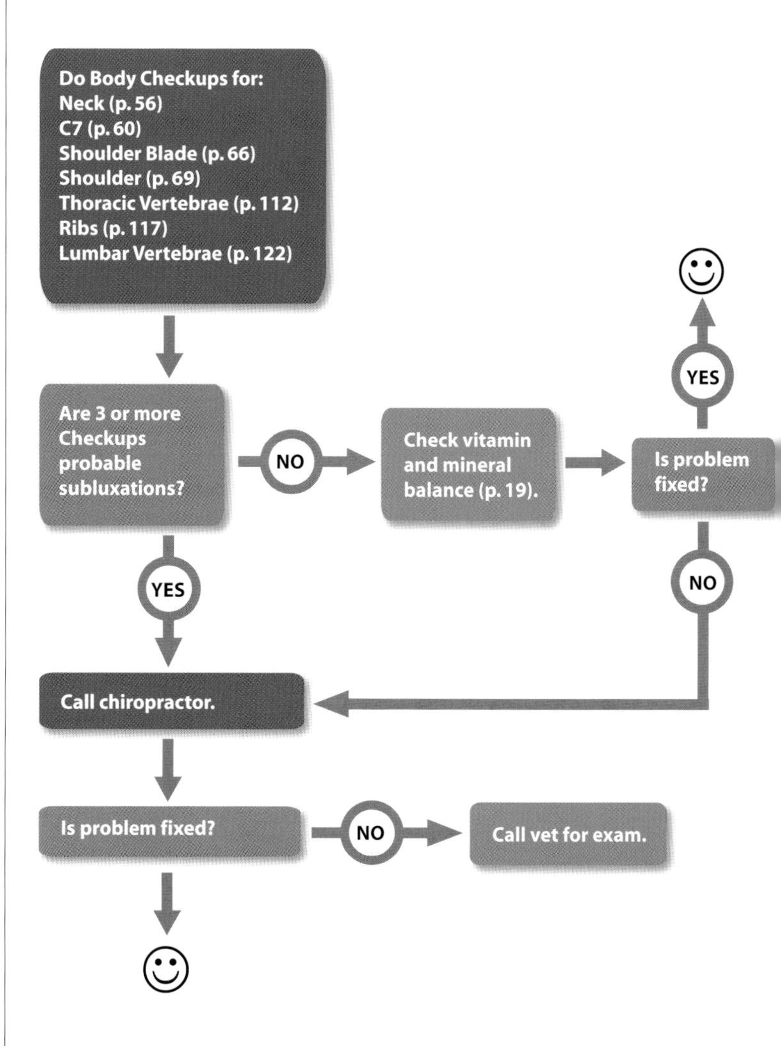

7. "GIRTHY"

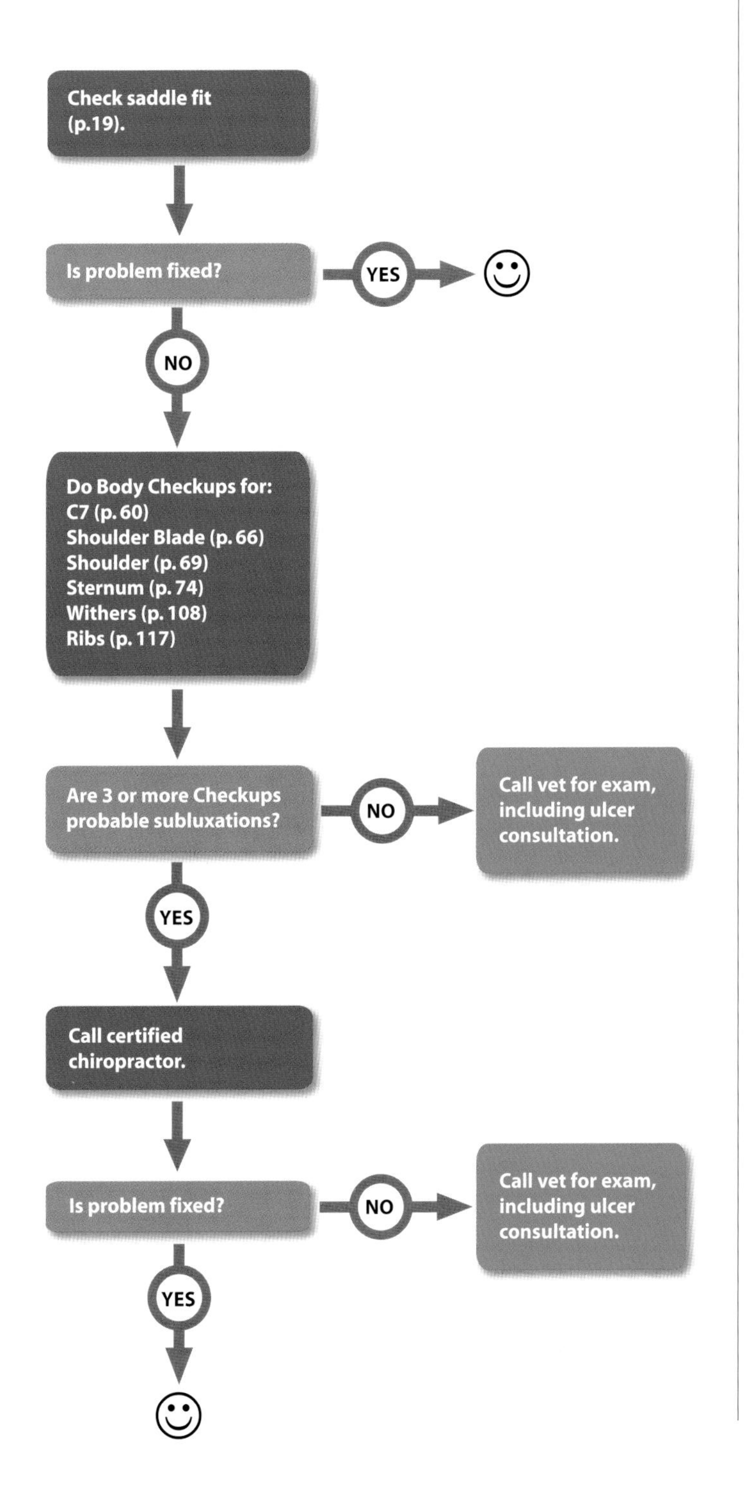

8. TRAVELS WIDE AND/OR DROPS SHOULDER ON TURNS

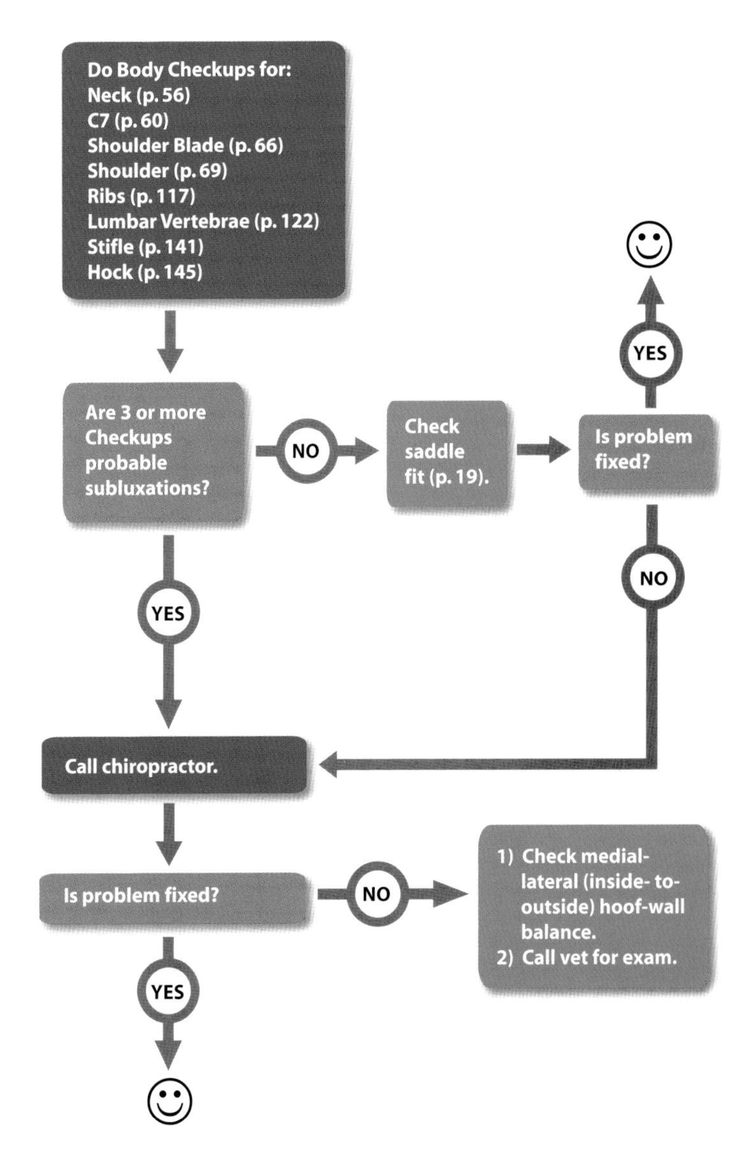

9. RIDER FEELS CROOKED OR SADDLE SLIPS TO ONE SIDE

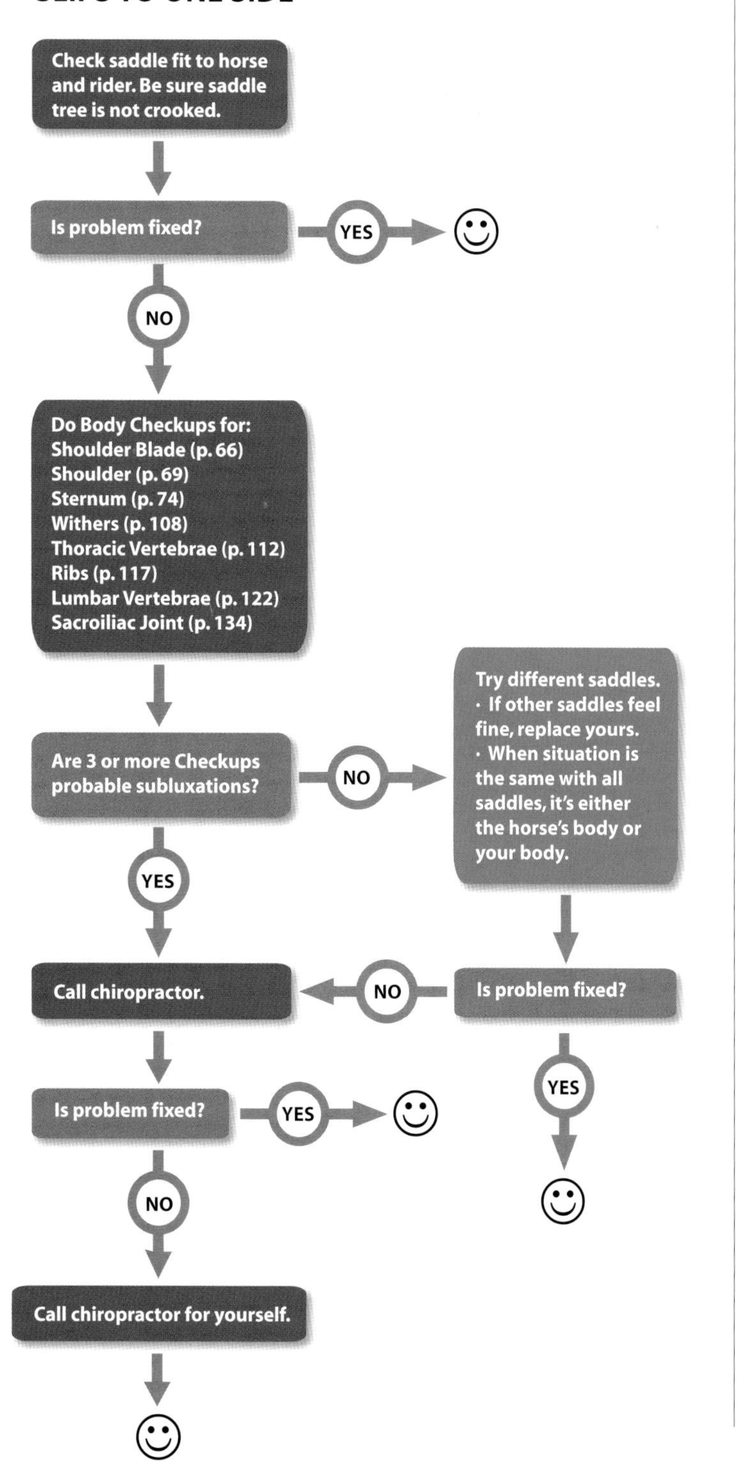

10. HORSE FEELS STIFF OR COLD-BACKED

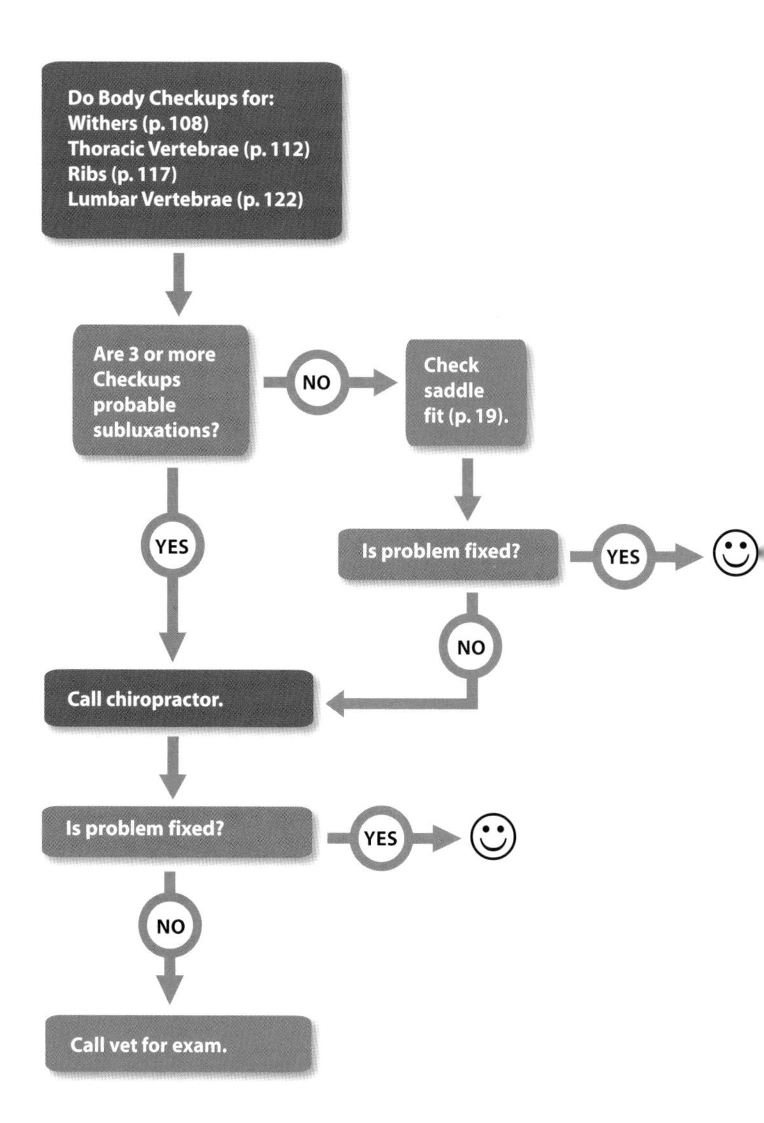

APPENDIX B

Comprehensive Complaints List

Atlas, recurrent subluxations of: Check *Occiput 48; TMJ 52*

Back, "cold-backed": Check *Withers 108; Thoracic Vertebrae 112; Ribs 117; Lumbar Vertebrae 122*

Back, muscles sore: Check *Thoracic Vertebrae 112; Ribs 117; Lumbar Vertebrae 122*

Back, muscles tight: Check *Thoracic Vertebrae 112; Ribs 117; Lumbar Vertebrae 122*

Bit, avoids contact with: Check *Atlas 44; Occiput 48; TMJ 52; Neck 56*

Body, reluctance to bend, one or both directions: Check *Neck 56; Withers 108; Thoracic Vertebrae 112; Ribs 117; Lumbar Vertebrae 122*

Body, stiff, may warm up to perform acceptably: Check *Withers 108 Thoracic Vertebrae 112; Ribs 117; Lumbar Vertebrae 122*

Breath, shortness of: Check *Sternum 74; Ribs 117*

Brushing, hypersensitive to: Check *Withers 108; Thoracic Vertebrae 112; Ribs 117; Lumbar Vertebrae 122*

Bucking/Crow-Hopping/Kicking Out, wants to, especially when ridden: Check *Thoracic Vertebrae 112; Ribs 117; Lumbar Vertebrae 122; Intertransverse Joint 126; Sacrum 130; Sacroiliac Joint 134*

Cantering/Loping, difficulty picking up, maintaining, or changing: Check *Atlas 44; Occiput 48; Lumbar Vertebrae 122; Sacrum 130; Sacroiliac Joint 134* (see also Leads)

Chewing food, difficulty on one or both sides of the mouth: Check *Atlas 44; Occiput 48; TMJ 52*

Circles, short-strided in front, one direction or both: Check *Shoulder 69; Elbow 77; Accessory Carpal Bone 84; Splint Bone 87; Sesamoid Bones 94*

Collection, difficulty with: Check *Atlas 44; Neck 56; Withers 108; Thoracic Vertebrae 112; Ribs 117; Lumbar Vertebrae 122; Sacrum 130; Sacroiliac Joint 134; Stifle 141; Hock 145; Tail Vertebrae 149*

Dental Problems, history of: Check *Atlas 44; Occiput 48; TMJ 52*

Direction, obviously prefers one over the other: Check *Atlas 44; Occiput 48; Neck 56; C7 60; Shoulder 69; Splint Bone 87; Sesamoid Bones 94; Ribs 117; Thoracic Vertebrae 112; Lumbar Vertebrae 122; Sacrum 130; Sacroiliac Joint 134; Stifle 141; Hock 145*

Downhill, reluctant to go: Check *Coffin Joint 102; Stifle 141; Lumbar Vertebrae 122*

Ears, afraid to have them handled/touched; ear-shy: Check *Atlas 44; Occiput 48; TMJ 52*

Ewe Neck, has: Check *Atlas 44; Occiput 48; Neck 56; C7 60; Withers 108*

Facial Expression, often indicates "I have a headache. Don't bother me." Check *Atlas 44; Occiput 48; Lumbar Vertebrae 122*

Farrier, difficulty holding up front feet for (see Front End, difficulty stretching)

Farrier, difficulty holding up hind feet for: Check *Lumbar Vertebrae 122; Intertransverse Joint 126; Sacrum 130; Sacroiliac Joint 134*

Fetlock, decreased flexion: Check *Accessory Carpal Bone 84; Sesamoid Bones 94; Fetlock 90; Pastern 98*

Focus and Concentrate, inability to: Check *Atlas 44; Occiput 48*

Foot, "clubby": Check *Shoulder 69; Elbow 77; Knee 81; Accessory Carpal Bone 84; Fetlock 90; Sesamoid Bones 94; Pastern 98; Coffin Joint 102; Ribs 117*

Foot, "high heel, low heel" syndrome: Check *C7 60; Shoulder Blade 66; Shoulder 69; Pastern 98; Coffin Joint 102; Hip Joint 137*

Foot, "tender-footed", especially if no obvious confor-mational cause: Check *Pastern 98; Coffin Joint 102*

Foot, hoof wall medial-lateral imbalance: Check *Elbow 77; Accessory Carpal Bone 84; Splint Bone 87; Sesamoid Bones 94; Pastern 98; Coffin Joint 102*

Foot, landing toe first: Check *Shoulder 69; Elbow 77; Knee 81; Accessory Carpal Bone 84; Fetlock 90; Sesamoid Bones 94; Pastern 98; Coffin Joint 102; Ribs 117*

Foot, tendency to grow excess heel: Check *Shoulder 69; Elbow 77; Knee 81; Accessory Carpal Bone 84; Fetlock 90; Sesamoid Bones 94; Pastern 98; Coffin Joint 102; Ribs 117*

Front End, lack of extension: Check *C7 60; Shoulder Blade 66,Shoulder 69; Elbow 77; Knee 81; Withers 108; Ribs 117*

Front End, reluctance to stretch legs: Check *C7 60; Shoulder Blade 66,Shoulder 69; Elbow 77; Knee 81; Withers 108; Ribs 117*

Gait Transitions, difficulty with: Check *Lumbar Vertebrae 122; Sacrum 130; Hock 145*

Haltering/Bridling, uncomfortable with: Check *Atlas 44; Occiput 48; Neck 56*

Head, reluctance to have it handled/touched; head-shy: Check *Atlas 44; Occiput 48; TMJ 52*

Hind End, difficulty with tracking up straight: Check *Lumbar Vertebrae 122; Intertransverse Joint 126; Hip Joint 137*

Hind End, uneven takeoff when jumping: Check *Lumbar Vertebrae 122; Sacrum 130; Sacroiliac Joint 134; Stifle 141; Hock 145*

Hocks, sore or other problems: Check *Lumbar Vertebrae 122; Sacroiliac Joint 134; Hip Joint 137; Stifle 141; Hock 145*

Impulsion, difficulty with: Check *Atlas 44; Neck 56; Thoracic Vertebrae 112; Withers 108; Ribs 117; Lumbar Vertebrae 122; Sacrum 130; Sacroiliac Joint 134; Stifle 141; Hock 145; Tail Vertebrae 149*

Interfering, front end: Check *Shoulder Blade 66; Shoulder 69; Sternum 74; Elbow 77; Splint Bone 87*

Jumping, reluctance to: Check *Knee 81; Fetlock 90; Sesamoid Bones 94; Pastern 98; Coffin Joint 102; Sacrum 130; Sacroiliac Joint 134; Stifle 141; Hock 145*

Knee, "bobbing" or "buckling over": Check *Elbow 77; Knee 81; Accessory Carpal Bone 84*

Knee, decreased flexion: Check *Knee 81; Accessory Carpal Bone 84*

Lameness, "phantom", front end: Check *C7 60; Sternum 74* (see also Strides, short in front)

Lameness, "phantom", hind end: Check *Sacrum 130; Sacroiliac Joint 134; Stifle 141; Hock 145; Tail Vertebrae 149*

Lateral Work, difficulty with front end: Check *Shoulder Blade 66; Shoulder 69; Elbow 77; Splint Bone 87; Sesamoid Bones 94; Fetlock 90; Withers 108; Hock 145*

Lateral Work, difficulty with hind end: Check *Lumbar Vertebrae 122; Sacrum 130; Sacroiliac Joint 134; Intertransverse Joint 126; Stifle 141; Hock 145; Hip 137; Tail Vertebrae 149*

Leads, counter-canters or cross-canters behind: Check *Sacrum 130; Sacroiliac Joint 134*

Leads, swaps out behind: Check *Sacrum 130; Sacroiliac Joint 134*

Leads, difficulty picking up, maintaining, or changing: Check *Atlas 44; Occiput 48; Lumbar Vertebrae 122; Sacrum 130; Sacroiliac Joint 134*

Standoffish/Non-Affectionate, frequently: Check *Atlas 44; Occiput 48*

Stiff, front end: Check *Neck 56; C7 60; Shoulder Blade 66; Shoulder 69; Knee 81; Fetlock 90; Pastern 98; Coffin Joint 102; Withers 108; Ribs 117*

Stiff, hind end: Check *Thoracic Vertebrae 112; Ribs 117; Lumbar Vertebrae 122; Sacrum 130; Sacroiliac Joint 134; Stifle 141; Hock 145*

Stifle, sore or other problems: Check *Lumbar Vertebrae 122; Hip Joint 145; Stifle 141; Hock 145*

Stirrups, rider feels one is short, but they're even: Check *Shoulder Blade 66; Shoulder 69; Sternum 74; Withers 108; Thoracic Vertebrae 112; Ribs 117; Lumbar Vertebrae 122; Sacroiliac Joint 134*

Stocking Up, in hind end: Check *Lumbar Vertebrae 122; Sacrum 130; Sacroiliac Joint 134; Hip Joint 137; Tail Vertebrae 149*

Strides, "off" in front, one foot or both: Check *C7 60; Shoulder Blade 66; Shoulder 69; Elbow 77; Knee 81; Splint Bone 87; Sesamoid Bones 94; Pastern 98; Coffin Joint 102; Withers 108; Ribs 117*

Strides, "off" in rear, one foot or both: Check *Ribs 117; Lumbar Vertebrae 122; Intertransverse Joint 126; Sacrum 130; Sacroiliac Joint 134; Hip Joint 137; Stifle 141; Hock 145*

Strides, short in front, one foot or both: Check *C7 60; Shoulder Blade 66; Shoulder 69; Elbow 77; Knee 81; Splint Bone 87; Sesamoid Bones 94; Pastern 98; Coffin Joint 102; Withers 108; Ribs 117*

Strides, short in rear, one foot or both: Check *Ribs 117; Lumbar Vertebrae 122; Intertransverse Joint 126; Sacrum 130; Sacroiliac Joint 134; Hip Joint 137; Stifle 141; Hock 145*

Tail, clamping: Check *Lumbar Vertebrae 122; Sacrum 130; Tail Vertebrae 149*

Tail, held to one side, either moving or at rest: Check *Lumbar Vertebrae 122; Sacrum 130; Tail Vertebrae 149*

Topline Muscles, difficulty developing: Check *Atlas 44; Neck 56; Withers 108; Thoracic Vertebrae 112; Ribs 117; Lumbar Vertebrae 122; Sacrum 130; Sacroiliac Joint 134*

Topline Muscles, difficulty using: Check *Atlas 44; Neck 56; Withers 108; Thoracic Vertebrae 112; Ribs 117; Lumbar Vertebrae 122; Sacrum 130; Sacroiliac Joint 134*

Tripping, regularly trips in front end, one foot or both: Check *C7 60; Shoulder 69; Knee 81; Fetlock 90; Pastern 98*

Tripping, regularly trips in hind end, one foot or both: Check *Ribs 117; Lumbar Vertebrae 122; Intertransverse Joint 126; Sacrum 130; Sacroiliac Joint 134; Hip Joint 137; Stifle 141; Hock 145*

Trot, prefers to over other gaits: Check *Sternum 74; Thoracic Vertebrae 112; Ribs 117; Lumbar Vertebrae 122; Sacrum 130; Sacroiliac Joint 134; Stifle 141; Hock 145*

Turns, short-strided in front, in one direction or both: Check *Shoulder 69; Elbow 77; Accessory Carpal Bone 84; Splint Bone 87; Sesamoid Bones 94* (see also Strides)

Turns, difficulty with: Check *Sesamoid Bones 94; Fetlock 90; Pastern 98; Coffin Joint 102; Stifle 141; Hock 145* (see also Body Bending)

Turns, drops shoulder, one direction or both: Check *Shoulder Blade 66; Shoulder 69; Sternum 74; Withers 108; Ribs 117; C7 60*

Turns, goes wide, one direction or both: Check *Neck 56; C7 60; Shoulder Blade 66; Shoulder 74; Ribs 117; Lumbar Vertebrae 122; Stifle 141; Hock 145*

Turns, holds shoulder out: Check *C7 60; Shoulder 69; Elbow 77*

Turns, trips frequently: Check *Elbow 77; Splint Bone 87; Fetlock 90; Sesamoid Bones 94* (see also Tripping)

Work, "long-and-low" difficulty: Check *Atlas 44; Neck 56; C7 60; Withers 108; Lumbar Vertebrae 122; Sacrum 130*

Work, inability to ("exercise intolerance"): Check *Sternum 74; Ribs 117*

About the Author

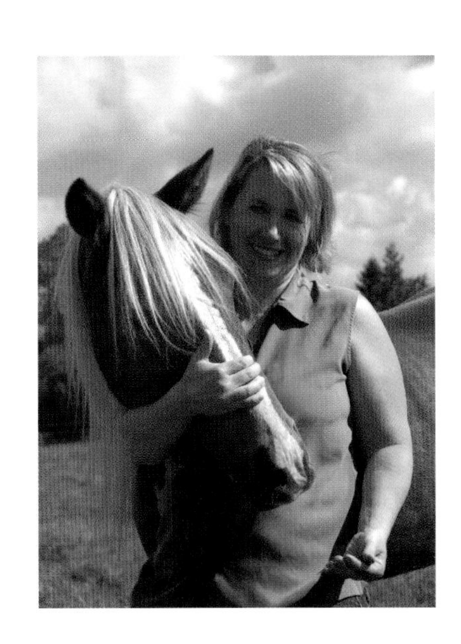

Dr. Renee Tucker received her Doctorate in Veterinary Medicine from the University of Tennessee in Knoxville, Tennessee. Although she grew up in a Chicago suburb and never owned a horse, this did not stop her from devoting her veterinary practice entirely to horses. Dr. Tucker added her Certification for Animal Chiropractic (CAC) in 1998, and her Acupuncture certification in 2000. She started her own private practice specializing exclusively in equine acupuncture and chiropractic work in 2000.

"How things work" has always been a question that Dr. Tucker has tried to answer. Prior to receiving her veterinary degree, she received her Bachelor's degree in Bioengineering. This unique combination of veterinarian and engineer has enabled her to create a special approach for helping owners help their horses. This approach combines her medical knowledge of equine health with her engineering background of simple, step-by-step problem solving.

Dr. Tucker currently resides with her two sons in Redding, California. She enjoys reading, cartoon movies, and dreaming of owning her own doughnut shop. Dr. Tucker invites you to contact her at renvet1@gmail.com, and via her website www.wheredoesmyhorsehurt.com.

Author Testimonials

"My Andalusian mare, Damsel, was in pain everywhere, and she could not round her back after months with the wrong trainer. A friend suggested Dr. Tucker and her gentle techniques. The results were stunning: Physically, my horse was pain-free, fast. The emotional results were equally huge. Damsel recognized I understood and cared about her pain and the depth of our bond expanded. Dr. Tucker's techniques will help any horse: This book explains how. Owners whose love for their horse(s) is both wide and deep will want a copy."
—Gail Wells-Hess, Portland, Oregon

"Dr. Tucker has worked on many of the horses out at my barn over the past years, and I have seen so much improvement in those horses. Not only soundness issues, but attitudes changed. Horses that were cranky (because they were in pain) are now happy to do their jobs! I really like the fact that Dr. Tucker uses a gentle method of chiropractic care, my horses really like it when she works on them, you can see the relief in their eyes!" **—JoLynn Turner, Ridgefield, Washington**

"I have a big, black (age 19 now) Trakehner, and he'll be showing Grand Prix again. When 'Eddy' came from Germany four years ago and Dr. Tucker first laid eyes upon him, she commented how his long back muscles were 'seized' from withers to loin. His body didn't make a natural curve from spine to tummy—the muscles stuck out like big 'dually' truck fenders. Dr. Tucker applied her chiropractic skills, and those 'fenders' vanished right before our eyes! Only at that moment did we both realize we should've taken 'before' and 'after' pictures, because anyone seeing them would instantly become a believer in the value of chiropractic for horses!"
—Joy Vartanian, Fox Island, Washington

"Dr. Tucker has been working on my horses for about five years. She has worked wonders. Her intuition and gentleness, along with her effectiveness, are quite miraculous. She has helped my animals immensely."
—Laura Cohen, Toledo, Washington

"I first met Dr. Tucker 12 years ago. In her, not only did I find a chiropractor but one who is a vet and knows the intimate workings of the horse and fully understands the suffering our show horses go through to do what they do. I was thrilled! Almost all my clients have had their horses seen by Dr. Tucker. I fully believe that she is a huge reason why in 10 years I only had one suspensory issue. I feel it was she who kept my horses that did have soundness issues going—and I've had more than one held together with 'duct tape and a prayer.'

"I will never forget one of the horses Dr. Tucker worked on in my barn—this horse came into my program and DID NOT EVER land on the left lead after a jump. I worked and worked with him to no avail. I convinced his owner to have Dr. Tucker look at him, and in Dr. Tucker's words, he was 'a disaster.' I knew then life was about to get better for him. The first day I rode him after she worked on him, with his owner standing there watching, he landed on the left lead after a jump and repeated it several more times. His problem had nothing to do with a training issue—he physically couldn't do it. At that moment, his owner was a made a believer of the importance of body maintenance for our equine athletes." **—Amy Ruge, Vancouver, Washington**

"I have lived and trained all over the United States, and I have never found anyone that so thoroughly helps my horses in training. Dr. Tucker has the highest integrity. She loves the animals she works on and they know it. She has taken old show stars that have been 'left for done' and allowed them to have new careers again and again. My own horses always fall asleep and drool when she works on them. I have never found a horse not improved from her work—she has been a huge help with backs and withers sore from years of bad saddle fitting. I would not be as successful as a trainer without Dr. Tucker on my maintenance team."
—Julia Kubicek, Battle Ground, Washington

"I am a lifetime horse owner, trainer, show person, and enthusiast. I was having trouble getting my horse Shadow (a 10-year-old Tennessee Walking Horse gelding) to flex on one side. I knew he was trying but something was holding him up. The trainer/clinician suggested I look into chiropractic care, but I must admit I was skeptical, having had bad experiences myself.

"At a recent equine expo, I found Dr. Renee Tucker's booth—a Veterinarian that specializes in a unique combination of chiropractic and acupuncture healing. I explained Shadow's symptoms and she told me to attend her demo on 'how to know when to call for an adjustment.' I showed up at the evaluation clinic and the horse scheduled wasn't available. So I offered to bring my horse Shadow to the ring for the demonstration. It was a great experience to learn how to evaluate my horse to see if treatment was truly needed. Poor Shadow was a very good example of what to look for in the poll (it was not level), the spine (it was stiff a third of the way up from the tail head), the ribs (were sensitive), the rear legs (had reduced flexion), and the shoulder. They were all stiff or out of alignment and it was easy to see this.

"Dr. Tucker agreed to stay late after the show and help Shadow and me. It was fascinating to see how she worked and how the horse responded with relaxation—and, I think, relief. I could see the results during the session as we were able to get suppleness in areas of the spine that didn't move during the demo and alignment in other areas. Dr. Tucker told me to give him a few days off, then resume riding.

"I noticed a difference right away as I watched Shadow move around in the pasture, relaxed and supple. But the really noticeable improvements were a week later when I really started riding. It was like a miracle (no joke). It made a huge difference in his performance, he was much more relaxed, not dropping his shoulder to the inside, and easily flexed both ways. I am overjoyed at this progress and feel relieved that my horse is more comfortable and moving better. However, I am also very humbled. I consider myself a very knowledgeable equine person but never thought to consider this type of care for my horse. I have a lot to learn each day and will always include Dr. Tucker in the care of my equine partners, even though it is a three-hour journey to see her.

"I think Dr. Tucker has a one-of-a-kind, holistic approach to care of the horse. I highly recommend her to any equine enthusiast, regardless of breed, discipline, or interests."**—Belinda Becker, Sultan, Washington**

"Dr. Tucker gets great results, and best of all, the horses love the process. When she is working, their head goes down, their eyes soften, and they melt under her touch. I would recommend Dr. Tucker's technique for an adjunct therapy for any horse with minor soundness issues."**—Natasha Lefkowitz, DVM, Portland, Oregon**

"I think this book should be a must-read for every horse owner. Dr. Tucker has put together information to help horse owners keep their horses happy and sound in their work. I know it has made a difference with all of my (many) horses!"**—Karol Rich, LMP, EBW, Battle Ground, Washington**

"I have been blessed in my life to have met a few people with truly remarkable healing abilities, and Dr. Renee Tucker is one of the best. I have so much to be thankful to her for...I have a 17-year-old Thoroughbred, and I could tell there was something that just wasn't right—he was not himself. Trainers said, 'Come on, make him do this,' or 'He is just being lazy.' But we were struggling. After trying various other therapies, changing my saddle, and double-checking the fit, still there was something off. Then a friend suggested Dr. Tucker. The results were profound—I watched my horse come back to being his old self. He was able to do what I was asking of him, and he had that engaged look about him, not so shut down.

"But what struck me the most were two things. Firstly, the 'feel' that Dr. Tucker has—she really 'senses' what the horse needs, from poll to tail. She works with the complete horse. And secondly, the adjustments held! I have never seen such big results with such gentle work. I can't begin to understand what she does, but am so inspired by the results I have seen."—**Lucy Metcalf, Portland, Oregon**

"My Friesian stallion had been experiencing trouble learning lateral movements. His refusal to move away from the right leg seemed to be very perplexing to everyone who worked with him. It was almost as if he was two completely different horses on the left versus the right side of his body. He had been imported from Holland at age three with no history of major falls or injuries, and with a clean extensive veterinary health check.

"A good friend suggested Dr. Renee Tucker to me. At our first appointment, she explained that my horse showed signs of a significant fall of some type, and the resulting misalignment had caused extensive muscle tightening and spasm. She spent a great deal of time and effort with both my horse and me explaining the issues involved, suggesting basic supplement changes that I could make to help him recover from his old injury and prevent further problems, and proving invaluable in helping me discover what I needed in an excellent saddle fit. Within three months, my horse's condition had completely resolved. More to the point, within the next six months he learned all the lateral movements including half-pass, developed a fabulous collected canter, and we started flying changes! What a difference it made to have my stallion balanced and comfortable in his body. I owe a great deal to Dr. Tucker's skillful assessment." **—Kathleen Carroll, Kelso, Washington**

Index

Page numbers in *italics* indicate illustrations.